THE
DIABETES
SOLUTION

THE
DIABETES
SOLUTION

How to Control Type 2 Diabetes
and Reverse Prediabetes Using
Simple Diet and Lifestyle Changes

JORGE E. RODRIGUEZ, MD

and Susan Wyler, RDN

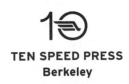

TEN SPEED PRESS
Berkeley

Published in the United States by Ten Speed Press, an imprint of the Crown Publishing Group, a division of Random House LLC, a Penguin Random House Company, New York.
www.crownpublishing.com
www.tenspeed.com

Ten Speed Press and the Ten Speed Press colophon are registered trademarks of Random House LLC.

   Library of Congress Cataloging-in-Publication Data

Rodriguez, Jorge E.
 The diabetes solution : how to control type 2 diabetes and reverse prediabetes using simple diet and lifestyle changes / Jorge E. Rodriguez, MD, Susan Wyler, RDN.
   pages cm
1. Diabetes—Popular works. I. Wyler, Susan. II. Title.
RC660.4.R63 2914
616.4'62—dc23
                        2014026487

Hardcover ISBN: 978-1-60774-616-4
eBook ISBN: 978-1-60774-618-8

Printed in the United States of America

Design by Betsy Stromberg

10 9 8 7 6 5 4 3 2 1

First Edition

CONTENTS

PART TWO

MANAGE YOUR DIABETES

INTRODUCTION

M Y FATHER WAS a closet diabetic. I always knew he had high blood sugar, but no disease was ever mentioned in the family. It wasn't until I was in the middle of writing this book that something clicked, and I asked my mom whether my dad had been diabetic. "He took insulin twice a day," she said. I was astonished. I am a physician, a specialist in internal medicine who should have known his father's medical history, but it wasn't until she divulged this information that it all started to make sense.

In his disease progression, my father was the stereotypical candidate for type 2 diabetes. During his youth he was a thin, baseball-playing, athletic, Errol Flynn look-alike—a very handsome, dynamic man. As he aged, however, he stopped exercising and became sedentary. He began to develop the midlife paunch common to so many men. When he was in his late forties he had his first heart attack. By the time he was sixty he had developed congestive heart failure, and he died of cardiac arrest within the year. Losing him broke my heart. My dad was one in a million, and twenty years later I still miss him very much.

As a physician, I know that more than 50 percent of diabetes sufferers end up dying of cardiovascular disease. But I also know that if we screen for the disease and catch it early, we have many tools to help reverse it while it is still in its incipient stage, which we call *prediabetes*. Once this condition has advanced to full-blown type 2 diabetes, these same tools and many medications are invaluable for lowering the elevated blood sugar that is the hallmark of the disease as well as helping to prevent or control long-term side effects.

I can't help but wonder how much of what happened to my father could have been prevented or put off for years if his diabetes had been treated earlier or if he had changed his lifestyle. The same can be asked about eighty million Americans who are living with type 2 diabetes, not to speak of the roughly twenty-five million who have the disease and don't know it.

Because diabetes develops slowly and doesn't hurt, far too many people are unaware they are suffering from this silent killer. Most of us would prefer to look the other way when it comes to dealing with an unpleasant health issue. Because screening is not mandatory, and many people skip their annual physicals, it's easy for blood sugar to creep up, along with blood pressure and weight, without any health care professional sounding an alarm. And not all doctors choose to discuss weight with their patients. A pity, because overweight and obesity go hand in hand with type 2 diabetes, which is why the disease is running rampant. I'd like to put a stop to that. It's our goal in this book to explain in very clear language not just what diabetes is and how it progresses, but more important, what can be done to control it. I don't want one more person to go through what my father suffered.

Treatment plans for type 2 diabetes or prediabetes must be individually tailored. Because I can't see all of you as patients, I've teamed up with colleague Susan Wyler, a registered dietitian in private practice who also teaches in the graduate nutrition department of the University of North Carolina at Chapel Hill. Together, we've created a comprehensive tool kit that offers the broadest possible range of information on type 2 diabetes. This holistic approach, based on the very latest in scientific research, is most effective because it helps you take charge of your care in partnership with your physician. Between the two of us, we are widely versed in medical treatment of type 2 diabetes as well as the lifestyle modifications that are most effective for controlling the disease: proper nutrition, weight loss, physical activity, stress reduction, and diabetes self-management education techniques—everything you need to halt your disease and prolong your life. All these factors add up to *The Diabetes Solution,* a compilation of medical treatments and lifestyle behaviors that have been proven in scientific studies to improve health in the present and prevent complications in the future. Chapter by chapter, throughout this book, we explain each of them in detail, one step at a time.

It's our fervent wish that you take this information and apply what is relevant to your life. We hope that the comprehensiveness and breadth of the advice will help you better understand your disease and how it can most effectively be treated. If this causes you to have a better dialogue with your health professional, then we have done a good job. Remember, no book can take the place of a doctor; use the information you find here to help yourself and to become a more educated patient. *The Diabetes Solution* is not meant to be a substitute for your doctor; it's meant to be an informative guide that will help you partner with your doctor for the very best results possible.

As a physician with more than thirty years of clinical experience, I have found that patients are much more likely to take their medications correctly or change their unhealthy habits if they understand why doing so is important. My main tool as a doctor is not medication, it is persuasion, and my most powerful weapon is scientifically proven truths. I know that when I explain, in clear, simple terms, just what diabetes is, what harm the disease can cause, and how we can stop the damage, you will do the right thing for yourself. I have faith in you. *The Diabetes Solution* is your biggest ally.

Throughout the pages of this book you will learn to understand what type 2 diabetes is, why it occurs, what damage it causes, and how you can prevent it. Together, Susan Wyler and I have devised a three-pronged attack: knowledge, medication, and lifestyle. Undoubtedly, if lifestyle changes alone can control your diabetes that is the best choice. But some people can't make the adjustments. They try to lose weight, but often fall back. Many just think about it. Soon months turn into years, and they are still obese. In the meantime, irreparable kidney damage or nerve damage may have taken place, just to name a couple of common complications of diabetes.

This really is a matter of life and death. If you can't change your lifestyle or your blood sugar remains high, medication is your best friend. I stress the importance of diabetes drugs, including insulin where needed, until you get the diet and lifestyle changes under way. To help you there, we've developed a whole range of suggestions to improve your health. But the crown jewel of this book is the Blood Sugar Budget, a balanced way of eating that represents the healthiest diet for almost everyone and the most effective way for those with type 2 diabetes or prediabetes to lower their blood sugar and lose weight. You'll be surprised how much good food awaits you.

The Diabetes Solution offers everything you need to know about type 2 diabetes and its precursor, prediabetes, neatly and clearly outlined. It is designed to be a tool that you can use practically, referring to it daily in conjunction with treatment recommended by your personal health care professional. I hope that *The Diabetes Solution* will inspire you, encourage you, and keep you on track. Here's wishing you a long and healthy life.

—Jorge E. Rodriguez, MD

PART ONE

KNOW YOUR ENEMY

CHAPTER 1

UNDERSTANDING TYPE 2 DIABETES

WE ARE AT WAR here on U.S. soil. Everyone knows the name of the enemy, but very few people can identify it, let alone describe what it looks like. I'm talking about the diabetes epidemic. At first it may seem like I am being overly dramatic; after all, it's *only* diabetes. That is part of the problem. Diabetes has become such a familiar word and popular media topic that we tend to underestimate its impact and take it for granted.

Well, try to ignore these facts. It is estimated that prediabetes and type 2 diabetes affect more than fifty million people in the United States and are directly responsible for more than 250,000 deaths per year. You thought I was exaggerating about being at war? Think again.

Here is another alarming statistic: diabetes is the seventh leading cause of death in America. And that rank should actually be higher, because more than half the people with diabetes actually die from cardiovascular disease, to which diabetes strongly contributes. But the staggering statistics of diabetes don't end here.

Type 2 diabetes is associated with both aging and excess body weight. As the population gets fatter and fatter and the median age climbs rapidly with the maturation of the baby boomers, this once relatively rare condition has turned into a full-blown epidemic. Plus, type 2 diabetes can affect anyone and potentially everyone. It does, however, favor certain populations. African Americans, Hispanics (excepting Cuban Americans), and Native Americans are at greater risk. Asians born in America have an elevated risk of diabetes, as well. Whether this is purely a genetic factor or more likely a combination of genetic tendency and lifestyle, especially diet, has not been fully established.

An epidemic is measured not only in the number of people it affects, but also in the amount of damage it causes. I have already mentioned how many people die from type 2 diabetes, but the number of people who suffer permanent health damage is also staggering. Damage to the kidneys from type 2 diabetes is the leading cause of end-stage renal disease in the United States. When the kidneys can no longer function properly, patients are forced into dialysis, filtering the blood through a machine three or four times a week. They have to follow a very strict diet, and if they are late in getting their regular dialysis, it can be very painful.

Am I trying to paint a very bleak picture just to scare you? No. But I am trying to paint a realistic picture so you can confront this disease early on while it's still very treatable. That is what distinguishes type 2 diabetes from so many other chronic diseases. You can manage it and prevent or mitigate future complications; but to do so, first you have to know whether or not you have it.

WHO, ME?

A few months ago a very prominent personality disclosed on a television interview show that he had diabetes. Initially I thought this was great because it would increase awareness about the illness. Instead, this person blew it off with a joke and basically stated that it was not a big deal and could be treated with diet and exercise; no medical intervention needed. This nonchalant attitude really put me off. Unfortunately, such blasé dismissal of the disease is not new, but with this book we do hope to teach people to take diabetes seriously.

I remember being an intern at the University of Miami. During those long nights we were on call, we would admit dozens of people who were critically ill. We would start patients on treatment for their illnesses, and we would also have to brush up and learn everything about their diseases, because early the next morning we would present the case to our attending professors. Not only was it imperative that we knew all the facts about their condition, but if we wanted to succeed with our supervising professors, we had to make sure we offered the correct treatment. This is how we were judged. This is how we become physicians.

I clearly remember the case of one woman who was obese, had signs of kidney damage, and kept complaining that her feet were numb. At the same time, she told me she had no preexisting conditions and was not taking any medications. When I presented my case to my attending physician, he looked at me a bit skeptically. My presentation did not make sense to him. When he went to see the portly woman, all he had to ask was one question that clarified the whole situation.

He looked at her calmly and asked, "Are you taking any injections?" She responded, "Oh, sure. Insulin for my diabetes." I was stunned. Not only did it look as if I had not been thorough, but also the patient was so matter-of-fact about her diabetes that she didn't consider it a disease. And she didn't consider her insulin a medication.

That is why we are writing this book. Not only is diabetes one of the most common diseases in the United States, but it is also one of the most misunderstood and ignored. The fact that you have chosen to read this book is a great start. It shows that you want to inform yourself. Whatever your connection to type 2 diabetes, I'm glad you're reading this book, because the disease is a silent killer that usually comes on gradually and in its early stages often causes no obvious symptoms. In fact, it's estimated that one in three people suffering from the disease don't even know they have it.

If high blood sugar hurt, type 2 diabetes would have been brought under control decades ago. But in its initial stages, *hyperglycemia*, or elevated sugar in the blood, is painless and may not display obvious symptoms for some time. Only laboratory tests will detect elevated blood glucose levels, and not everyone is screened regularly. Many people lack health care coverage, and of those who do have it, not everyone goes for a general physical every year.

The good news is that if identified, type 2 diabetes is highly responsive to diet, exercise, and stress reduction. How many chronic diseases can be controlled through lifestyle modifications? I want you to pay attention to the advice that follows because it really is effective. And the same techniques used to lessen the effects of diabetes once it has developed can also help prevent it in the first place. I'm so excited about what we have to say that I'm afraid I'm going too quickly already. Let's start with the basics.

WHAT IS DIABETES?

My simple definition of diabetes is this: *diabetes is a disease characterized by abnormally high levels of blood glucose due to the body's decreased production of or decreased sensitivity to insulin.*

This may not make a lot of sense right now, but by the end of this book you will know what diabetes is, what causes it, what kinds of damage it does, and most important, what you can do to stop its progression or cure it completely. So pay attention and learn as much as you can, because you know what they say: keep your friends close and your enemies even closer. The best thing you can do to conquer this manageable chronic disease is to understand clearly how it works and how you can attack it most efficiently and effectively. Putting your head in the sand is not a good strategy.

If you've already received a diagnosis of type 2 diabetes from your doctor, chances are you had one of the following reactions. As I've said, in its early stages, this insidious disease has subtle symptoms and produces no pain. So if you're not really familiar with diabetes, your response may be very offhand:

- Okay, so what? If I ignore it or stop eating so many sweets, it will go away.
- I don't want to take any more pills, no matter what.
- Maybe there is something I can do that doesn't involve medication. I've got a lot of time to deal with this.
- It doesn't bother me and I don't have any symptoms, so I really don't care.

For those who are familiar with the disease because it runs in the family or who have a friend who is diabetic, it's a very different story. Their reaction may be one of sheer terror, especially if they've seen the disease leading to amputation of a foot or major limb. Fully 60 percent of leg amputations in the United States are attributed to complications from diabetes. Such fear can motivate, but it can also be paralyzing. The key to healing power is knowledge.

There are basically two main types of diabetes. We physicians in our infinite wisdom have decided to call them type 1 and type 2. Susan and I debated for a long time whether this book should be about both types of diabetes. In the end we decided to focus on type 2 diabetes, not because we think it is a more important or more serious disease than type 1 diabetes, but because it affects many more people; 95 percent of people diagnosed with diabetes have type 2. And this acquired type stands a much greater chance of being controlled with measures other then just medications. Type 1 and type 2 diabetes are quite distinct from each other.

Type 1 Diabetes

Type 1 diabetes is an autoimmune disease. In other words, for whatever reason, the body's own immune system has "turned" on itself and destroyed some of its own cells. In the case of type 1 diabetes, very specific cells found in the pancreas, called *beta* cells, have been destroyed. The job of the beta cells is to produce a hormone called *insulin*, which is required for the body to use the carbohydrates we eat as a source of energy. Without insulin, the sugar floats aimlessly in the blood, causing damage to small blood vessels.

People with type 1 diabetes usually are diagnosed when they are very young. They also tend to have much higher blood sugar levels than people with type 2 diabetes and are much more likely to go into a state of what's called *ketoacidosis*. In diabetes, the body cannot efficiently use glucose as an energy source, and so instead it uses fat. That may sound like a great idea at first, but unfortunately ketones are very harmful to the body; they are acidic and cause quick damage to our organs. Type 1 diabetes can also create extraordinarily high levels of blood glucose, which may cause someone to fall into a high blood sugar coma. Though diet and exercise may help, almost without exception type 1 diabetes must be treated with insulin.

Type 2 Diabetes

In very simple terms, type 2 diabetes is a condition in which the pancreas does not produce enough insulin, or, especially when paired with obesity, the insulin that is being produced is not doing its job. In the latter case, the body does not respond to the insulin signal because too much abdominal fat "stands in its way." We call this *insulin resistance.*

In a body that is functioning normally, carbohydrates in food are broken down into glucose—the body's primary source of fuel for producing energy. Glucose is then carried by the blood to cells throughout the body. With the help of insulin, cells absorb glucose from the blood and use it to make energy. In people with type 2 diabetes, however, no matter how much "sugar" they eat, their cells don't receive the fuel they need to produce energy.

What does it actually mean when your doctor gives you a diagnosis of type 2 diabetes? Well, most immediately, it signifies that you have abnormally high blood sugar. There is extra sugar circulating in your bloodstream, a higher concentration than the normal range of 64 to 99 milligrams per deciliter. So-called "prediabetics" register in a higher range of 100 to 125 mg/dl. A concentration of 126 mg/dl or higher indicates that diabetes is present.

It's the irony of this disease that although its hallmark is too much sugar in the blood (thus high blood sugar), the glucose that is floating around cannot get into the cells where it is needed. So even though people with type 2 diabetes may eat a lot, perhaps even too much, they are not fueling their body. Therefore, fatigue, lethargy, and hunger are common symptoms.

As we've said, type 2 diabetes is by far the most common type, accounting for about 95 percent of all diabetes. Type 2 diabetes usually occurs in adults, which is why it used to be called *adult-onset diabetes*. One reason there are an estimated more than twenty-five million cases of this disease in adult Americans over twenty is that this type of diabetes is strongly associated with obesity. In adults sixty-five years and older, it is estimated that almost 27 percent have diabetes and 50 percent have prediabetes, the milder precursor of diabetes, which we explain in detail in chapter 3.

Type 2 diabetes and overweight/obesity are inextricably linked. The country's obesity epidemic has opened the doors to type 2 diabetes on a scale never before imagined. What is even scarier is that the full effects, both physical and financial, of the present diabetes epidemic will not be felt for decades.

Though it's true that only 15 percent of overweight or obese people will go on to develop diabetes, when you multiply this by the 68 percent of the population that is overweight, plus include the 50 percent of those obese individuals with a body mass index (BMI) of 30 or higher, the numbers are huge: close to fifty million. With the aging and fattening of America, these statistics are expected to rise sharply in the near future.

And with so many teens and even children overweight and obese, we're seeing more and more diabetes in this age group, which we health care professionals find shocking. In the past, the only kind of diabetes we used to see in young people was type 1, or so-called "childhood diabetes." The times they are a-changin'—and not in a good way.

Unlike type 1 diabetes, which can eventually result in total depletion of the body's supply of insulin and often causes tremendous thirst and dramatic weight loss, type 2 can fester silently for years, doing internal damage to many organs without anyone knowing. Eventually, when blood sugar levels are high enough and the body can no longer compensate, symptoms much like those of type 1 diabetes will appear. I like to say that the most common symptom of type 2 diabetes is *no* symptom at all, because people can have the disease for years and be oblivious of the damage it is doing. But if symptoms do arise they may include one or more of the following:

- Persistent tingling in the legs and feet
- Unquenchable thirst
- Excessive urination
- Fuzzy vision
- Chronic fatigue
- Unusual weight loss or weight gain

Caught early while it is still technically prediabetes, the disease is easily manageable and even reversible for many people. (Chapter 3 explains everything you need to know to combat prediabetes.) But if the elevated blood sugar (hyperglycemia) has not been detected and has been allowed to run uncontrolled for years, type 2 diabetes can be devastating. Damage to the tiniest of blood vessels over time invariably leads to any number of complications, resulting in medical problems. These problems can shorten life by as much as nine years. They include, among others:

- Retinopathy: damage to the retina that can lead to blindness
- Kidney failure, leading to the need for dialysis
- Neurological damage, leading to early dementia or cognitive impairment
- Increased tendency toward atherosclerosis, or so-called hardening of the arteries, resulting in heart disease and stroke. In fact, more than 50 percent of people with diabetes eventually die of cardiovascular disease.
- Neuropathy: microscopic blood vessel damage and death of nerve cells, most commonly in the feet, which can result in undetected and fast-growing infections leading to foot and leg amputations
- Erectile dysfunction: an inability to get and/or maintain an erection due to both poor blood circulation to the penis and decreased sensation

Every organ of the body, including the heart, is susceptible to damage from diabetes. Even prediabetes takes its toll. Many men complaining of erectile dysfunction are unaware that it can be caused by high blood sugar. Likewise, lack of sexual response in women can be attributed to diabetes.

HOW TYPE 2 DIABETES IS DIAGNOSED

Because damage is occurring long before a person with diabetes has symptoms, early screening is essential for prevention of complications. And if detection happens early enough, many cases of prediabetes can actually be reversed. Catching type 2 diabetes early is the key. We want to diagnose it while the beta cells are still able to produce insulin. If after diagnosis you can get your weight down, improve physical activity, and reduce the body's inflammation, then you stand an excellent chance of improving insulin sensitivity and reducing your blood glucose levels.

There is a measure of what your average blood sugar has been over the past few months. It is called the A1C level (more about this in the next chapter). Some sugar molecules travel through the blood by attaching to the hemoglobin that carries oxygen in the red blood cells. Because we know red blood cells live for about three months, measuring the glucose attached to them gives us an average of how much sugar has been in circulation over the past several months. It is one of the ways we diagnose diabetes. Keeping the A1C at or below certain levels has been shown to prevent permanent damage.

I know that I am throwing a lot of new terms at you. But bear with me. I will continue to explain as we go along. I just want you to know that there is hope in reversing the damages of type 2 diabetes. Early diagnosis gives you a tremendous advantage, but the most important message is to get tested, no matter your age or health; there is always a chance to act on what you learn.

With prediabetes, the ideal goal is to achieve an A1C level below 5.7 percent; healthy people have an A1C from 4.5 percent to 5.6 percent. For people already diagnosed with type 2 diabetes, an A1C of less than 7 percent is the goal; some doctors strive for even tighter control of 6.5 percent. As usual in medicine, there is some controversy about these guidelines. Keeping the A1C more toward the lower number is controversial, because it can result in hypoglycemia, or low blood sugar. Hypoglycemia can cause fainting and cardiovascular episodes. However, we're seeing less hypoglycemia with newer medications. And as more studies are done, more physicians believe that the lower the blood sugar, the better—and as soon as possible, in terms of preventing irreversible blood vessel damage.

Over the years, the official ideal A1C levels and another measure called the random fasting glucose numbers have been lowered by the American Diabetic Association as well as by the World Health Organization and the AADE (American Association of Diabetes Educators). That means that standards for prescribing lifestyle changes and medications have become more urgent. It's *not*, as some would like to believe, that doctors benefit from writing more prescriptions. It's that study after study has shown that because the damage to tiny blood vessels and nerves occurs much earlier, it is *very* important to control high blood sugar levels as early as possible— yes, even if this means taking medication very early on.

However, major studies have shown over and over that although medication may be necessary to get a grip on the disease, diet, exercise, and other lifestyle adjustments are even more powerful than the most commonly prescribed drug, metformin. People who receive individual nutrition counseling and education about diabetes self-management techniques fare much better than those who don't, by all standards of measure.

TYPE 2 DIABETES AND NUTRITION

As you can tell by now, type 2 diabetes is an immensely complex disease. It is strongly associated with overweight and obesity, but some thin people have it, too. Much research points to some kind of systemic inflammation as the underlying cause of the damage created by type 2 diabetes. Many scientists are also exploring environmental triggers for the disease. Arsenic, for example—which is found in some chickens, in rice and processed rice products (like rice milk, rice breakfast cereals, and even baby cereal), in grape juice and apple juice, and in drinking water—has shown a direct relationship with the occurrence of type 2 diabetes. That's one reason why we are so adamant that if you can afford to eat organic and pure whole foods, it's the best way.

Type 2 diabetes is acquired largely through poor diet, lack of physical activity, and weight gain. What does that mean? It means that unlike many other debilitating chronic diseases, type 2 diabetes is largely preventable and, if caught early and treated aggressively, potentially curable or at least highly controllable.

Because the potential cure for type 2 diabetes is diet and exercise, it is essential that you understand some basic nutrition. Most people insist that if you have type 2 diabetes, you have to give up all sugar and sweets. Wrong—though you certainly want to reduce the amount of sugar and refined carbohydrates in your diet significantly. Others feel that you have to eat as little as possible and almost starve yourself throughout the day. Wrong again. But before we even get into that, you need to understand the relationships among sugar, glucose, carbohydrate, and starch.

All our food is made up of three major components—carbohydrates, fats, and proteins—along with tiny amounts of vitamins, minerals, and other trace elements that enhance health.

- Carbohydrates are the body's primary source of fuel; every cell in the body can burn glucose for quick energy. Carbohydrates are also essential for the health of our nervous system and the function of our organs, and vital for gut health and regularity. Most of what we call fiber is composed of carbohydrates.

- Fats provide the most concentrated form of energy, which is why they are used for storage. Fat is burned for fuel especially when we're exercising over time, but it has other purposes often downplayed in our "anti-fat" culture. Fat cushions our organs. We cannot absorb our fat-soluble vitamins—A, E, D, and K—without it. And fats maintain the health and suppleness of our cell membranes, where molecules are exchanged and chemical "messages" are transmitted. They are vital for normal growth and development.

- Protein can be used for energy as necessary if carbohydrates are not available, but its primary function is growth of tissues, repair of any damage to the body, and preservation of muscle mass. Enzymes and hormones are proteins that direct all the functions of the body. And proteins bolster the immune system.

Each of these large groups of macronutrients has a different chemical composition. But we don't eat chemistry, do we? We eat food. Understanding how these substances translate into real grocery store ingredients and how they affect our bodies can help anyone with type 2 diabetes or prediabetes chose what to eat to control blood sugar. That is one of the ultimate goals of *The Diabetes Solution*.

If you've been diagnosed with type 2 diabetes or prediabetes, most doctors and health educators will urge you to cut back on carbohydrates, especially so-called refined carbohydrates, which are higher in pure starch and low in fiber. "Eat a low-carbohydrate diet," they'll say. A dietitian or nutritionist who helps you plan your diet in more detail will recommend eating them in combination with fats and protein, and preferably in high-fiber dishes. Some will tell you to avoid all white foods: white bread, white rice, biscuits, mashed potatoes. They'll encourage you to choose whole grains, which contain a mix of soluble and indigestible fibers as well as protein, vitamins, and minerals, with a smaller proportion of starch. They may talk about glycemic index and glycemic load. What's the difference? Why is it okay to eat some foods and not others? And what is a carbohydrate anyway? Understanding a little bit of science will help you realize that "carbs" per se are not to be feared, but they do need to be controlled. That means choosing the right carbohydrate in the first place and eating it at the right time and in the appropriate amount.

In a nutshell, think of carbohydrates as fuel and yourself as a very sophisticated engine. Carbohydrates provide us with energy that comes from the sun—literally. It is the electromagnetic energy contained in sunshine, processed through the chlorophyll in plants that takes carbon dioxide from the atmosphere and water from the soil and creates the molecules made up of carbon, oxygen, and hydrogen that we call *carbohydrates*. Talk about solar energy!

In its most basic form, a carbohydrate is what we think of as sugar—it tastes sweet on the tongue. What's a little more confusing is that the sugar molecule *glucose* forms the base of all starches as well. Many carbohydrates, strung together in different patterns, create starches: the foods we know as flour, bread, pasta, rice, corn, and other grains. These are what we call complex carbohydrates. Hey, it doesn't take a rocket scientist to figure out how that name was derived.

Any food with starch in it is made of long chains of glucose strung together in both straight lines and complex matrices and webs. The digestion of sugars and starches—both carbohydrates—begins in the mouth. Chewing and tasting trigger release of moisture from the salivary glands, which contain an enzyme, amylase, that quickly begins to digest carbohydrates even before they reach the stomach.

Starches may not taste sweet in the mouth, but as soon as they hit saliva and then encounter stomach acid and are digested, which happens very rapidly, they break down into their component sugars. A starch (complex carbohydrate) will dissolve into the most basic sugar so it can be absorbed into the bloodstream. So, to paraphrase Shakespeare, "a carbohydrate, by any other name, will not taste as sweet," but it's still all the same to the body.

In truth, there are many different sugars, but most of those we eat can be reduced down to glucose—a single-molecule sugar—which is the fuel our bodies run on, like gasoline in a car's engine. Glucose is also your brain's favorite food. We need this energy not just to run or play tennis or hike; we need it so we can breathe, so our muscles can contract and our cells can reproduce—so we can live. It's these carbohydrates that have the greatest immediate effect on the amount of sugar in our blood.

Because life happens every moment but we eat only occasionally, we need a way to retain carbohydrates for energy between meals. Your body stores the carbohydrate you are not using in your muscles and in your liver in the form of *glycogen,* a sort of spare energy source that can be called upon quickly or during fasting. Once you have reached the maximum amount of glycogen that can be stored, the other excess calories are stored in the form of fat all over your body. (And you know I'm not kidding when I say *all* over your body.) The reason for this is that fat is much denser than carbs. You can pack almost twice as much energy into the same space. Fat contains 9 calories per gram, whereas both protein and carbohydrates hold only 4 calories per gram. If we didn't have fat, we'd be as big as houses. I know, hard to believe that fat is actually making us look skinnier.

You've heard of too much of a good thing? Anyone who is overweight or obese is taking in too much energy and storing too much fat. Ironically, many people who are overweight and obese are suffering from what we call "undernutrition." They're taking in far too many calories, the extra portion of which is converted into more fat, but they are getting too few vitamins, minerals, and fiber as well as other valuable chemicals we get from plant-based food sources, which help us metabolize our food properly.

With diabetes, the biggest part of the calories, or energy, goes to waste because while it is ingested, the body doesn't utilize it. Without enough insulin secreted by the pancreas or with too much resistance to the insulin that is produced, the sugar just hangs around in the blood, and the cells are deprived of the energy they need. Then the body senses low energy, and matters become worse because this stimulates the liver to produce glucose and pump it out into the bloodstream, where it simply raises blood sugar levels even higher. So simply eliminating carbs from your diet is not the solution. In fact, the healthiest way for someone with diabetes to eat is to avoid *excessive* carbohydrates but to take in a moderate amount evenly throughout the day. To understand why this is beneficial, you need to understand the role of a couple of very important hormones: insulin, which we've already introduced, and glucagon.

Normally, the blood sugar level is maintained within a healthy range by a pair of hormones: *insulin*, which we already explained is produced in the beta cells of the pancreas, and *glucagon*, which is produced in the *alpha* cells of the pancreas. Insulin is released in response to the presence of glucose in the bloodstream. Glucose appears in the blood after we eat. This stimulates the release of insulin, which ushers the sugar into the cells and lowers blood glucose. Because we need energy to live, during short periods of fasting (eight hours or less) between meals if necessary, the liver makes a certain amount of glucose, too. It is glucagon's job to stimulate the liver to make glucose. Insulin and glucagon work as a team. In a normally healthy body, when the blood sugar is high, the pancreas releases insulin. When the blood sugar is low, the pancreas releases glucagon. Type 2 diabetes develops chiefly as a result of abnormal functioning or production of insulin.

It's insulin's purpose to usher that glucose from the bloodstream into the cells. Actually, you can think of insulin as a gatekeeper: it unlocks a gate that opens a channel through which glucose flows into the cells, where it's burned like the body's gasoline. This combustion produces the energy we need to run, play, breathe, and even think. Without that energy, or without enough of it, your cells are virtually starved and cannot function properly. Before the advent of modern pharmacology and the discovery of insulin in the pancreas in the early 1920s, people with type 1 diabetes would simply die in a matter of months.

Visualize your body's energy system as a subway train. It has to run twenty-four hours a day. Think of the people boarding the train as glucose. They make everything happen in the city. Without the people, everything comes to a halt. Your blood flows through arteries and veins like the train through its subterranean tunnels. People enter the train through gates at the stations. If the turnstiles don't move or the human traffic becomes too congested, no one can get on the train or only a few can enter every time the door opens. Meanwhile, the crowd backs up in the station and up the stairways. Nothing proceeds the way it's supposed to. The city comes to a slow but sure stop.

Insulin makes sure the turnstiles open so people can reach the trains, so the energy in your blood can enter the cells. But if there is not enough insulin to open the gates, or there is too much traffic, the insulin cannot reach the gates, and blood sugar builds up in the vascular system. This buildup causes permanent damage to the blood vessels.

The first step in curing a disease is to understand its cause. Even though we have a long way to go in knowing all the intricacies of diabetes, science has established an excellent foundation.

IS THERE A CURE FOR DIABETES?

The scientific effort to find a cure for diabetes is in its infancy. We're still learning to understand the disease. We do know that the most effective treatment is very individualized. Diabetes is not a one-size-fits-all disease. To the contrary, each individual needs to have a treatment plan uniquely tailored to him or her, by a doctor and a dietitian.

A holistic approach is best. This means combining medical care under the guidance of a physician, who can monitor glucose levels and prescribe proper pharmaceuticals, and nutritional guidance with a registered dietitian nutritionist, who can recommend appropriate diet, physical activity, stress reduction, and natural supplements. Together they can devise a program to reverse prediabetes or control type 2 diabetes, dodging the very serious, life-threatening complications that arise over time if blood sugar is not managed properly.

That's why we feel *The Diabetes Solution* is so important. It can give you the tools you need to reduce the chances of the disease occurring in the first place, to reverse prediabetes, or to manage type 2 diabetes if you have already been diagnosed. Understanding the nature of your illness and what you can do about it will empower you. *The Diabetes Solution* offers a comprehensive plan to battle this ever-more-common disease by starting at the beginning and taking you—the patient, potential patient, or family member of the patient—step by step through everything you need to know to cope with and potentially conquer this deadly but unnecessary illness. The first step is to understand how doctors test you to see whether you are at risk for the disease or already have it.

CHAPTER 2

SCREENING FOR TYPE 2 DIABETES

MY BROTHER, COUSINS, and I emigrated from Cuba when we were children. When we arrived, my brother, Amaury, was only six months old; I, on the other hand, was a much more mature two years old. We were lucky. We learned to speak English and Spanish at the same time. I honestly can't tell you which one I learned first. As best I can recall I learned them both simultaneously. Being bilingual was not a conscious decision; it just happened. So when all the young cousins would get together, we would switch effortlessly between both languages, sometimes creating our own third language: Spanglish. We could talk as easily about "Los Beatles" as we could about "Mami's delicious *arroz con pollo*," her Spanish chicken with rice. It seemed natural to us. We were thrilled with our linguistic dexterity. Our parents and grandparents, however, were not as pleased.

As you can imagine, my parents and grandparents had a much more difficult time learning English. Spanish had been the only language they knew. It was especially difficult for my grandmother Ofelia. She complained that she was losing touch with her grandchildren because she could not communicate with them. So one day she put her foot down. She told us in no uncertain terms that we were to speak only Spanish at home. She figured we would get all the English we needed at school and on the streets. While we were under her roof we had to speak one common language: Spanish.

I tell you this story because with diabetes, the same will be true for you. Having diabetes is a whole new world, filled with a whole new language. In order for you to conquer your diabetes, you must first understand this strange language being spoken around you. You must understand the meaning of these new words and tests. Perhaps now you can sympathize a bit with my grandma's and my parent's plight. At first they didn't know the difference between "lightning" and "lightening," but eventually they conquered the language—and so will you. That mastery allowed them to reach their goals and become very successful—and it will for you, too.

We are determined to arm you with this new language because knowledge is power. Some studies suggest that as much as one-fourth of the U.S. population may have undiagnosed diabetes—a staggering number. This is not just because the disease has no symptoms in the early stages. It is also because the language of diabetes is foreign to most of us. If the first step toward treating diabetes is finding out whether you have it or not, the first step toward finding out is learning the language.

Now, for your first language lesson.

DEFINING DIABETES

You already know that diabetes is the state of having excessive glucose in your bloodstream, due either to the underproduction of insulin or the insensitivity of your body to the insulin it produces. The end result is the same: constantly high levels of blood glucose that cause damage to many of the body's organs. But how do doctors determine whether someone has diabetes? There are three blood tests used by physicians to detect diabetes, any one of which alone is sufficient to make the diagnosis.

There are a few professional organizations of diabetic experts whose opinions are so respected that once they analyze the most current research information and reach certain conclusions, their recommendations quickly become the gold standard of care. One such group is the American Diabetes Association (ADA). In 2014, the American Diabetes Association revised many of its definitions and recommendations. The definition of diabetes, however, has stayed fairly standard. Diabetes is currently diagnosed in one of three ways. You only need one of the three to be positive to be given the diagnosis of diabetes.

- A Fasting Plasma Glucose (FPG) greater than or equal to 126 milligrams per deciliter (mg/dl). For this test, fasting is defined as not having had any caloric intake (not eaten *anything*) for at least eight hours before the test.

- An Oral Glucose Tolerance Test (OGTT) in which the two-hour plasma glucose is greater than or equal to 200 mg/dl. The glucose used for the test is 75 grams of glucose dissolved in water.

- A Hemoglobin A1C (Hgb-AIC) greater than or equal to 6.5 percent. This test can be drawn at any time. You do not have to be fasting.

"Que significa eso?" my grandmother would ask. "What does it all mean?" Let's look at these tests that define diabetes, one by one.

Fasting Plasma Glucose

Plasma is the liquid component of blood in which the red blood cells, white blood cells, and so on swim. The Fasting Plasma Glucose (FPG) test, which is done with a simple blood draw, is the measure of your blood sugar after you have not eaten for at least eight hours. It has been found that after eight hours any individual's blood sugar should be below a certain level. Everyone, that is, except a person with diabetes.

After eight hours of fasting, someone without diabetes' plasma blood glucose level will *always* be below 100 mg/dl. Always. No exceptions. Many of my patients with an elevated FPG try to explain their result away by stating that they had a large meal the night before the blood test. Sorry, folks: it doesn't matter whether you ate a whole pecan pie or a wheelbarrow full of doughnuts the night before. If you are not diabetic, your body will be able to metabolize that high glucose load within the eight hours, and your plasma level *will* be below 100 mg/dl.

That is why it is so important to not cheat and to take this test when you have indeed been fasting. If you followed instructions and fasted for at least eight hours before the blood test, the result is valid. If you did eat within those eight hours (even that coffee with sugar or that little bite to tide you over), first of all, you are disobedient, and second, it completely invalidates the test. Completely. No correct conclusion can be derived. It must be repeated. So don't cheat on this one. If you do, it could cause you to mistakenly be labeled a diabetic when you don't have the disease.

The FPG should never be higher than 100 mg/dl. Never. If it is, you have diabetes or prediabetes. The range between 100 mg/dl and 126 mg/dl is considered prediabetes and must be taken as seriously as diabetes, because organ damage is probably already occurring. Many physicians advocate placing patients with prediabetes on a low-carbohydrate diet and exercise program to lower their blood glucose. I am one of those physicians. (Read more about prediabetes in chapter 3.)

If your blood plasma glucose is equal to or greater than 126 mg/dl in a Fasting Plasma Glucose test, you have diabetes. No doubt about it; end of the discussion. Many of my patients who receive such a result cannot believe it. They doubt the result because they have no "symptoms." They usually want me to repeat this test. The truth is, many people with diabetes do not develop the classic symptoms sometimes for decades. Early in the course of the disease, the damage that is being done is silent; it is what we call "microvascular." Microvascular refers to the smallest blood vessels throughout the body, especially those in the eyes, the kidneys, the nerves, and the genitals. By the time you can feel that damage, it is already extensive. Think of a body with diabetes as a house with termites. The termites are destroying the house long before the first wood beam collapses.

If the FPG result is positive, it is appropriate to repeat the test to make sure it was correct. Almost all doctors order a second confirmatory test. If you have an abnormal FPG, your physician may even order one of the other two defining blood tests.

Fasting Plasma Glucose is an adequate screening test. It is good at diagnosing someone who has obvious or advanced diabetes because there is no way to disguise a high plasma glucose. But the FPG is a bit weak in diagnosing someone with prediabetes or borderline diabetes. I have had many prediabetics and even diabetics who in preparation for their appointment with me ate very "cleanly" for the couple of weeks prior to their FPG test. In other words, they may have suspected that they had elevated blood sugar and for those two weeks they ate the correct amount of calories per day and exercised regularly. When their FPG was done, their test was below 126 mg/dl. If a physician still suspects a person may be diabetic, one of two other diagnostic tests should be performed.

Oral Glucose Tolerance Test

As I just explained, it is sometimes difficult to have patients follow all the specifications needed to obtain an accurate FPG. I've had many patients come for their *fasting* blood draw after drinking a coffee with cream and sugar. After I question them, the usual response is, "Oh, I didn't know I couldn't *drink* anything either. The instructions just said don't *eat* for eight hours." Imagine a doctor's frustration. Especially when all we are trying to do is diagnose someone early enough to avoid diabetes' long-term complications. One reason the Oral Glucose Tolerance Test (OGTT) was conceived was to try to avoid such mishaps.

OGTT is not really simpler to perform. You still have to fast for at least eight hours. Plus, you must hang out for at least two hours while a few blood samples are drawn. But what is great about it is that it is reproducible. If a patient has a doubt about the diagnosis, it can be run again and more likely than not the result will be identical. What is being tested here is how quickly your body metabolizes a set amount of glucose that you are asked to drink. Your body will metabolize this the same almost every time—unless you have lost a considerable amount (some say at least 5 percent) of your body weight between tests.

After decades of studying diabetes, medical science now knows what constitutes a normal insulin response to a premeasured amount of consumed glucose. In other words, if I give ten healthy people a premeasured amount of sugar to eat, we know the average amount of sugar that should be in the blood thirty minutes after it was eaten. We also know how much sugar should be in the blood two hours after the glucose is eaten. We know how quickly it should be cleared from the blood and the highest acceptable level that someone's plasma glucose can reach. That is the basis for the OGTT.

A patient is told to eat normally for days or weeks before the OGTT. On the morning of the test, the patient needs to be fasting from all food and liquids. A baseline blood glucose is then obtained. After this, the patient is given a premeasured solution of glucose syrup to drink. It *always* contains 75 grams of glucose. That is the standard and never varies. Some of the older OGTTs required that blood be drawn at thirty minutes, sixty minutes, and two hours after the consumption of the glucose. However, for diabetes screening all that is really needed is the baseline glucose measurement and the two-hour post-consumption glucose measurement. It is with the result of the two-hour plasma glucose measurement that we decide whether someone has diabetes.

Quite simply, if two hours after the consumption of 75 grams of glucose your blood serum glucose is 200 mg/dl or greater, you have diabetes—no ifs, ands, or buts. We can get more information from this test, too. If two hours after the drinking of the sugar solution your blood serum glucose is below 200 mg/dl, but between 140 mg/dl and 199 mg/dl, you have what we call *impaired glucose tolerance.* Impaired glucose tolerance is another name for *prediabetes.* This means your body was very slow in metabolizing the sugar you were given. Imagine this happening every time you ate. Your sugar would be at an unacceptably high level almost all the time. This level of sugar floating around your blood has been proven to be dangerous. It is silently damaging many of your organs, even though technically its concentration doesn't fall into the diabetic range.

Any result under 140 mg/dl is considered nondiabetic. What I most like about the OGTT is that it is reproducible—if the instructions are followed correctly. However, the OGGT can still be fallible, depending on whether the patient truly fasts before the test. Is there any test that is relatively "patient proof"? The hemoglobin A1C is a close as it gets.

Hemoglobin A1C–Glycated Hemoglobin

Our blood is full of thousands of chemicals and compounds—enzymes, proteins, fats, red blood cells, and white blood cells, just to name a few. They travel in this river of liquid plasma, bouncing around aimlessly. Each of these blood components has unique electrical charges on the surface. Much like pinballs bouncing around until they find that hole that is a perfect fit, our blood components bounce around until they find matching opposite electrical charges. This match takes compounds to areas where they are needed. These matches can create a very long-lasting or at times permanent bond. Such a bond occurs between the glucose in our blood and the red blood cell (hemoglobin).

It was discovered in 1958 that blood glucose binds to the surface of hemoglobin. The result was called hemoglobin A1C (or just A1C, for short). Glucose forms a very tight bond with hemoglobin that can last for the life span of the red blood cell (an average of three months). Imagine the surface of your red blood cells being covered by sugar. The percentage of the surface that is covered with glucose molecules is very telling of how well your body metabolizes sugar. By 1969 it was discovered that people with diabetes had an increase in their A1C. Makes sense, doesn't it? The less you are able to take that sugar into the cells throughout the body and metabolize the glucose, the more glucose will remain floating in your blood. The more sugar you have bouncing around in your blood, the more will bind to the surface of your red blood cells.

By 1976 it was clear that the A1C could be used not only to diagnose diabetes but also to monitor how successful a patient was at controlling his or her blood sugar. Many studies have shown an almost perfect correlation between a diabetic's A1C and what his average daily blood sugar has been over the past three months. In other words, if over the past three months your daily blood sugar has been 150 mg/dl, your A1C may be 7.0 percent. That means there has been enough glucose floating around to bind to 7.0 percent of the surface of your blood cells. But if your average daily blood sugar has been 200 mg/dl, there has been so much glucose floating around your blood that it could easily have covered 8 percent of your red blood cell surfaces. In other words, your A1C would be 8.0 percent.

To visualize this, think of a nice red juicy strawberry as one of your red blood cells. Think of thick rich chocolate as your blood glucose. For argument's sake, let's say that having a glucose of 140 mg/dl will fill a glass one-quarter of the way up. Now imagine dunking that strawberry in that glass. How much chocolate is covering the surface of the strawberry? That chocolate is your A1C. If your average glucose were 200 mg/dl, then the glass would have more chocolate, and when you dunked your strawberry, the surface would have more chocolate and likewise your A1C would be higher.

It is important that every minute of the day we have a normal blood sugar, because any time it is not normal, there is damage to your organs. With the A1C measurement, we now have a tool that allows us to see how well a person has really done in controlling her blood sugar over the previous few months without having her take a blood glucose sample every morning. The patient doesn't have to fast. She doesn't have to drink a certain amount of sugar syrup. We can simply draw a blood sample, and it doesn't matter whether she is fasting or not.

The American Diabetes Association has defined an AIC greater than or equal to 6.5 percent as indicative of diabetes. This test can be repeated again for confirmation, but it is usually conclusive.

If an A1C result is found to be between 5.7 percent and 6.4 percent, that person is diagnosed as prediabetic. Remember, although it is not full-blown diabetes, prediabetes is still a very serious condition and should not be taken lightly.

The A1C is useful not only for identifying diabetes. I find it most useful in determining whether a patient is truly adherent to his lifestyle change or whether a treatment change is actually helping. Remember, the higher your daily blood sugar has been over the prior weeks, the higher your A1C is going to be. Most studies suggest that the A1C is measuring the average daily glucose concentration over the previous four weeks to three months.

Other studies show that you can see improvements in the A1C within as little as twenty days after starting a new regimen.

The A1C test is not perfect, however. It has its limitations. If a person has another disease that causes the red blood cells to die more quickly than the usual three-month life span, the A1C may appear artificially low. For example, sickle cell anemia, G6PD deficiency, or an allergic reaction to other medications are some of the illnesses that cause early cell death and thus a misleadingly low A1C. On the other hand, deficiencies in B_{12} or folate may produce abnormally high levels of A1C. Be sure to make your physician aware of any other health issues you may have or supplements you are taking when you have your A1C tested. It may be very important in interpreting the results.

This chart helps show you exactly what your A1C means. For example, if your A1C is 9 percent, your average daily blood glucose level has been 212. That is *very* high. However, if after three months of diet and exercise you have been able to lower it to 7 percent, that is a very successful treatment regimen.

A1C Correlation with Mean Daily Plasma Glucose							
A1C (%)	6	7	8	9	10	11	12
Mean Plasma Glucose (mg/dl)	126	154	183	212	240	269	298

An increase in blood sugar, and therefore in A1C, increases the risk of long-term complications, such as coronary artery disease (leading to heart attacks), strokes, kidney failure, erectile dysfunction, neuropathy (loss of sensation), and gastroparesis (slow emptying of the stomach), just to name a few. A study of close to fifty thousand patients showed that diabetics with an A1C of greater than 6.5 percent had an increased rate of death when compared with nondiabetics and people with lower A1Cs.

Another series of trials showed that for approximately every 0.1 percent drop in A1C, the risk of developing long-term complications from diabetes decreases by 3 percent. In other words, if you drop your A1C by 1 percent (and maintain it there), you could theoretically decrease your risk of blindness, kidney failure, or erectile dysfunction by 30 percent. It's obvious that maintaining a low A1C is the ultimate goal of diabetes therapy. But how low is low enough? And how low is too low?

Let me start off by saying that every case is individualized. Some people get low blood sugar, or hypoglycemia, too often to try and maintain a very low A1C. In hypoglycemia there is not enough glucose in your blood to "feed" your muscles or your brain. You feel dizzy and clammy and could easily pass out. Therefore, maintaining a low A1C may be very dangerous, because if you skip a meal or work out too hard, that may be enough to send you over the line and into hypoglycemia. Imagine getting hypoglycemia while driving a car. It can be very dangerous indeed. Fortunately, the treatment is very easy: drink a juice that is very high in glucose. Orange juice works great. In a pinch, any piece of candy will do just fine. But it's better to avoid needing that fast treatment in the first place.

Some patients with diabetes may be so ill, and the damage already done to their body so extensive, that the risk of becoming hypoglycemic is too great. Plus, the damage has already been done, and keeping a very low A1C is not going to help much. In those cases there is no point in trying to keep very strict control of the A1C (below 6 percent). A slip into hypoglycemia could be a death blow and not worth the risk. In those patients whose diabetes is very advanced, I prefer the A1C to be between 6 percent and 7 percent.

In general, for most people, keeping the A1C at 7 percent or lower has been shown to reduce microvascular complications (neuropathy, kidney failure, and so on). And if you implement this soon after being diagnosed, the macrovascular complications, especially critical for heart disease, may also be avoided. Less strict guidelines for A1C (less than 8 percent) may be appropriate for patients, especially older adults, who get too many bouts of low blood sugar and become dizzy or pass out.

On the other hand, if a patient is young or recently diagnosed with diabetes or has no signs of complications, maintaining the A1C at less than 6.5 percent is a must. Because less damage has been done by this point, it is very important to be as aggressive as possible in lowering the A1C— assuming, that is, there are no significant bouts of low blood sugar. In other words, if you are a recently diagnosed diabetic without evidence of organ damage, lower your A1C to 6.5 or below to prevent organ damage. You need to strive for that low A1C.

All this information may seem daunting. But the bottom line is this: if you are diabetic and otherwise healthy, try and keep that A1C between 5.5 percent and 6.5 percent. But if you have too many bouts of hypoglycemia, or already have organ damage from years of untreated diabetes, an A1C between 6 percent and 7 percent suffices. As always, be sure to ask your doctor what A1C he or she feels is right for your state of health.

A1C is a very valuable tool. It is easy to measure, because all that is required is a blood test that can be drawn whether the patient is fasting or not. It has quickly become the gold standard in determining whether a certain diabetes therapy is working and whether you are really following your diet and lifestyle changes. A1C is both a screening test and an ongoing tool to see whether your current regimen is being successful. The FPG and OGTT have too much variation to be good tests in assessing ongoing success. Get to know what your A1C is; it could save your life.

WHEN TO SCREEN FOR DIABETES

Now that we know which tests are used to diagnose diabetes, this raises the question: who should get screened? First, anyone who has obvious symptoms of diabetes should go see her physician and alert him or her of her concern. By the time someone has the classic symptoms of out-of-control elevated blood sugar, the disease is quite advanced. Among these advanced symptoms are:

- Marked increase in urination
- Weight loss
- Blurry eyesight
- Persistent numbness of the hands or feet
- Erectile dysfunction
- Leg ulcers that do not heal
- Infections that take longer than usual to heal
- Heart attack
- Stroke

Kidney disease is another long-term complication of diabetes, but it usually does not cause symptoms until there is almost complete kidney damage. Short of a blood test to measure the kidney's ability to filter the blood, there may be no identifying signs.

My real concern is not so much the people who have symptoms, because most of them will eventually go to a doctor to get some answers. I am more concerned about the tens of millions of Americans who have

HOW IS LOSING WEIGHT A SIGN OF DIABETES?

Let me address something here that very often confuses people. Type 2 diabetes is associated with obesity and being overweight. Some people even simplify the matter and say that obesity causes type 2 diabetes. Usually the obesity comes first, followed by the diabetes. It is the state of being overweight, especially fat around the midsection, that contributes to the body being less sensitive to the insulin that is made. So let's follow this to its natural conclusion.

If you are overweight or obese, you are more likely than a normal weight person to become diabetic. Studies have shown that by a very intricate mechanism, the excessive storage of fat actually changes your body's ability to allow insulin to function properly. Thus, your body will not be able to use a portion of the carbohydrates that you consume. Those calories are going to waste, floating aimlessly in your bloodstream. It's as if you hadn't eaten them at all. So what happens then? Your blood sugar goes way up and your weight goes down, because those calories are not getting used; they are just floating in your bloodstream and eventually urinated out of your system. So, if you are an overweight person and *without trying* you begin to lose weight and urinate more than ever, you may be becoming diabetic. It's quite an efficient—but highly dangerous—way of losing weight.

diabetes and prediabetes who go undiagnosed because they have no symptoms. It is estimated that up to one-fourth of the total population of the United States may have undiagnosed diabetes. That is staggering. At least seventy-nine million Americans may not know they have diabetes as they sit down to enjoy a good old-fashioned piece of apple pie or chug-a-lug a liter bottle of cola.

If you ask me, everyone over the age of forty years old should be screened annually with a fasting blood glucose test. This is just my own opinion; much more scientifically based guidelines have been reached than the ones I reached from my own medical experience. But I am actually not too far from the recommendations. Mathematical models show that beginning screening at age thirty, independent of risk factors, is highly cost-effective in preventing or at least slowing down the development of future diabetes complications. Keep in mind, diabetes costs the health system a great deal: some estimates put it as high as $175 billion a year. As the population becomes more obese and the risk goes up, it only makes sense to screen sooner rather than later.

SCREENING PATIENTS WITH NO SYMPTOMS

Because tens of million of American go about their daily business without knowing they have diabetes, it is important we have guidelines to determine who is most likely to have undiagnosed or "silent" diabetes. The American Diabetes Association has summarized the scientific data and reached the following conclusions. Screening for diabetes and prediabetes

BODY MASS INDEX

Before I proceed with the recommendations for diabetes screening, there is one more phrase that I must add to your diabetes vocabulary: Body Mass Index, or BMI. BMI is basically a tool that estimates what proportion of a person's body is composed of adipose tissue (or fat). The BMI formula divides a person's weight by her height squared in metric measures. There are far better ways of assessing body composition, but they are expensive and inconvenient. Even though this is a rough estimate, it works well for most adults. Children hold a lot more water in their bodies, so BMI is not an accurate measure of their composition. And athletes with a lot of muscle, which is heavier than fat, may have an elevated BMI number but actually be a healthy weight. If you are a 5'2" woman and you weigh 150 pounds, your BMI is 27.4, and you are overweight. If you are a 5'10" man and weigh 220 pounds, your BMI is 31.5 and you are technically obese. This may seem ridiculous to some. In my opinion we have gotten so used to being overweight and seeing others who are overweight that we now consider it normal. You can easily calculate your BMI by going online and finding a BMI calculator. All you have to do is plug in your height and weight.

Many studies have been done that have correlated someone's BMI to the risk of heart disease and other obesity-associated illnesses. It has been established that a normal BMI ranges from 18.5 to 24.9 kg/m^2. Being overweight is defined as having a BMI between 25 and 29.9 kg/m^2. Obesity is defined as having a BMI equal to or greater than 30 kg/m^2. It is estimated that more than two thirds of Americans over twenty years of age are either overweight or obese. That number is staggering. Being overweight or obese and having type 2 diabetes go hand in hand. So indirectly, BMI gives us one more screening tool to use.

should be considered in an adult of *any* age who has a BMI greater than or equal to 25 kg/m^2 and who has one or more of the following risk factors:

- Physical inactivity
- First-degree relative with diabetes (mother, father, sibling, and the like)
- High-risk race/ethnicity (African American, Asian American, Latino, Native American, Pacific Islander)
- Previously delivered a baby weighing greater than nine pounds
- Previously diagnosed with gestational diabetes
- Hypertension (blood pressure greater than or equal to 140/90 mm Hg off therapy or anyone on hypertension medication)
- HDL cholesterol level less than 35 mg/dl
- Triglyceride level greater than 250 mg/dl
- Polycystic ovarian syndrome (PCOS)
- A1C greater than or equal to 5.7 percent
- Severe obesity
- History of cardiovascular disease (heart disease)

Because age is a major risk factor for diabetes, everyone should be screened beginning at age forty-five, even if they don't exhibit any of these risk factors.

HOW OFTEN SHOULD YOU BE SCREENED?

It is important that we stay honest about our health. The bottom line with these recommendations is that people who are overweight and have other health issues are the ones who have the most to lose by developing diabetes. So just because you were tested for diabetes once and the results were normal does not mean that you do not ever have to be screened again. As a matter of fact, it is recommended that if screening results are normal, testing should be repeated *at least* every three years. If the initial screening results were consistent with prediabetes, then screening should be done yearly. I cannot emphasize too strongly that diabetes is a silent killer that destroys vital organs slowly but surely. The only real way to slow down or halt this damage is to diagnose and treat it as soon as possible. Denial is your biggest enemy.

WHEN IS INTERVENTION RECOMMENDED?

Studies have shown that early intervention can decrease the rate at which high-risk individuals develop type 2 diabetes. As a matter of fact, this same research proved that lifestyle modification programs are very effective. Indeed, they can reduce by a whopping 58 percent the chance of developing diabetes in three years. Remember that statistic next time you are walking around the block or slowly jogging on the treadmill or forgoing a piece of pie in favor of a beautiful piece of ripe fruit. If you think diet and physical activity make no difference, think again. Some studies even show that early on, lifestyle modifications are even more effective than medication. The ability to control diabetes is yours. Your health is in your hands. But when is the best time to start treatment for diabetes?

If you have been diagnosed with diabetes, the time to start medication is, without a doubt, right now. The information is also fairly clear for people who have prediabetes: they should start a lifestyle modification program with several set goals at the time of diagnosis. This is covered thoroughly in chapter 3.

Lifestyle modifications begin with:

- A weight loss program to lose 7 percent of current body weight
- An increase in physical activity to at least thirty minutes a day, which can be divided up into multiple shorter exercise periods totaling thirty minutes

Diagnosed prediabetics should also be screened for other risk factors that contribute to heart disease, specifically high blood pressure and high cholesterol, immediately. And if they smoke, every effort should be made to stop. Remember, the major complication of diabetes is heart disease. It does very little good to control your blood sugar if you don't control the other risk factors, especially cigarette smoking!

Medication should be started immediately in anyone with prediabetes who also has at least one of the following characteristics:

- BMI greater than or equal to 35 kg/m^2
- Younger than sixty years of age
- Women with prior gestational diabetes

As you'll see in chapter 5 on medication, the drug of choice here is metformin. For these high-risk people, the combination of metformin *and* lifestyle changes reduces the incidence of progression to diabetes by 50 percent over those using medication alone. Quite impressive, if you ask me.

ONGOING MONITORING

If a patient of mine with type 2 diabetes is *not* on insulin, I monitor him with the A1C test sometimes as his only monitoring test. If we are trying a new medication, I check his A1C every three months and make any necessary changes at that time. If he is on a stable regimen, and nothing has changed in his health, I check his A1C only every six months.

It is acceptable to check the A1C less frequently because oral medications cannot be changed as easily as insulin dosages. You can change the amount of insulin you inject from day to day depending on the blood sugar and see an immediate effect. Not so with oral medications. It usually takes weeks before you see the effect on the blood glucose caused by changing the dosage of an oral medication. So I personally do not see a need to do daily finger stick glucoses if you are on pills to treat type 2 diabetes. I find that I can get a great idea of how well a patient is following her medication and lifestyle regimens easily and quickly by doing a periodic A1C. Plus, the test can be done in the office at the time of the office visit without the patient having to fast.

However, other physicians disagree and prefer for the patient to monitor his own blood sugar at home with a finger stick test or come in for a fasting blood sugar. Their rationale is that even though oral medication dosages should not be changed frequently, if a patient has daily blood sugars that are elevated, that serves as a warning. The patient can then immediately start modifying his food and/or exercise regimen. These doctors may have a point. But I find that if someone is new to medications, checking his A1C every three months until we have established the best regimen for him is sufficient.

The American Diabetes Association formally recommends that:

- The A1C test be performed at least two times a year for patients who are meeting their treatment goals and on a stable regimen
- The A1C test be performed every three months for patients whose therapy has been changed or who are not meeting their treatment goals

The ADA's recommendations seem to be similar to how I practice medicine. Recommendations are just that; they are not laws. Taking recommendations and fitting them into a patient's lifestyle is the art of medicine. There is often no one right way of doing things, though there are definitely many wrong ways of doing things. In the case of a diabetes regimen and monitoring, tailoring for the individual is crucial. For example, the busy executive or the stay-at-home mom have different time constraints from the full-time student. Their ability to check their blood sugar on a daily basis will be different. The lawyer and the day laborer have different budgets for food. All of these variables (time, money, and willingness) need to be taken into consideration when creating a medical and lifestyle plan for treating type 2 diabetes.

Now that you are better informed, you can better advise your physician what might work for you. This is much more likely to be successful now that you are both speaking the same language.

Being thrown into a situation in which you don't understand the language can be very scary. It must feel like that when you first go to a doctor's office and she starts talking about diabetes and A1Cs and fasting blood glucose. We doctors mention words and tests that you have never heard of before—until now. I hope this chapter has given you tools to understand our diabetes language. You don't always have to know the whole language to get by. You just have to know the right words. (My grandma will attest to that!) Now that you know some of the words, you understand enough to know that early diabetes is silent. You also know that the best way to prevent the very damaging long-term effects of diabetes is to diagnose it early and treat it aggressively. You also know now that it isn't just about starting a treatment; it is also about monitoring that treatment regularly to make sure it continues to work for you. You know a lot!

In the words of my grandmother: *"Felicidades. Ya sabes."* ("Congratulations. Now you have the facts.") Use that knowledge to get and stay healthier.

CHAPTER 3

UNDERSTANDING PREDIABETES

PREDIABETES IS ESSENTIALLY a precursor to diabetes. It's a condition that signals that your body is either in a state of insulin resistance or in the beginning stages of decreased insulin production. This means the pancreas may still be producing normal amounts of insulin, or it may be slowing down. But in either case, the insulin that is produced is not as effective as it should be in clearing glucose from the bloodstream. Your blood sugar has started to rise. Although it hasn't increased enough to call it diabetes, the rise may be significant enough to cause damage to your micro blood vessels. And it is estimated that, without treatment, 20 percent of people with prediabetes will develop type 2 diabetes within five years.

As noted in the previous chapter, when you have a diagnosis of prediabetes, it means that your fasting plasma glucose test results fall above normal levels but below the range for type 2 diabetes. This measurement is between 100 and 125 (remember that a normal result falls within a range of 55 to 99, with a measurement of 83 being squarely on the money, and 126 and higher being an indication of type 2 diabetes). In terms of glycated hemoglobin, or A1C (see page 26), a test that gives a broader impression of how much glucose on average has been circulating in the bloodstream over the past several months, prediabetes is indicated by a percentage range of 5.7 to 6.4, whereas type 2 diabetes registers 6.5 and higher.

Prediabetes is extremely common. A 2010 study from Emory University estimated that one in twelve Americans has both blood sugar high enough to qualify as prediabetes and other risk factors that suggest the use of metformin would be helpful. As of 2012, it was estimated that 35 percent of U.S. adults twenty or older would qualify as prediabetic. Again, that represents *seventy-nine million* people. Fully 50 percent of adults aged sixty-five and older have prediabetes, which has huge implications for the cost of Medicare.

Yet according to federal and state health surveys, fewer than 10 percent of U.S. adults with prediabetes report being given a diagnosis. This means either they've lived with the condition without being screened, or their health care professional did not fully understand how damaging even slightly elevated blood sugar can be and what a difference lifestyle changes can make. Prediabetes is an alarm to act *now* and to act decisively.

Sometimes putting a label on a condition is helpful; other times it's scary. I've seen a diagnosis of prediabetes provoke both reactions in my patients. The truth is, knowing you have prediabetes is upsetting because the label tells you that you do indeed have a real medical problem and greater risk of progressing to type 2 diabetes. But at the same time, being diagnosed can be beneficial because it identifies a condition that can be improved and potentially reversed.

Indeed, what is most encouraging about prediabetes is that, if it's caught early enough, in some cases blood sugar can not only be controlled, but also knocked down to normal levels. Whether this cure is permanent or represents only a slowing of progression to diabetes is open to debate and, in most cases, can be known only with time. But even without medication, some people can make lifestyle changes that actually reverse the condition. These changes include losing weight, exercising regularly, getting enough sleep, and relieving stress. Once your glucose levels come down to normal and stay down, you can lead a life without medication. Of course, ongoing proper nutrition and physical activity are essential to staying healthy.

Some people diagnosed with prediabetes will eventually progress to type 2 diabetes. These patients, who cannot totally reverse their condition, may well have a small genetic twist that over time slows production of insulin in the pancreas or interferes with the response to the insulin that is produced. But although these people cannot be completely cured, the same techniques that reverse prediabetes will slow the progression of full-blown diabetes, minimizing the need for medication for as long as possible and retarding or even preventing the many complications that may occur with the disease later in life.

As with type 2 diabetes, if you have prediabetes, it doesn't matter how much energy you take in or how much you eat: not all of the calories are made available to fuel your body. That's why people with prediabetes often feel sluggish and fatigued. Persistent hunger and unexplained weight loss—no matter how much you eat—are a couple of symptoms of diabetes.

DIAGNOSING PREDIABETES

In addition to testing your fasting plasma glucose numbers (see page 23) and your glycated hemoglobin (A1C; see page 26), the other test used to diagnose prediabetes is the oral glucose tolerance test (OGTT; see page 24). All three of these tests can determine whether someone has developed prediabetes.

These prediabetes glucose numbers are not arbitrary. They are low enough to indicate that your pancreas is still working, with the beta cells producing insulin, but high enough to suggest they are not making quite enough insulin or that something is preventing the insulin produced from acting properly. Prediabetes means the hormone is present but its message is not getting across. Either the signal is not being heard or it is too faint to be effective. Because the insulin is not acting properly, the glucose, or energy, from your food is not reaching the cells. You're running on low, and too much sugar is lingering in your bloodstream.

THE PREDIABETES-BODY WEIGHT CONNECTION

Given that more than 70 percent of the population is overweight or obese, and excess adipose tissue is associated with diabetes, it's not surprising that nearly seventy-nine million people in the United States have prediabetes. It's estimated that fully 50 percent of older adults suffer from this condition. Most of the people I diagnose with prediabetes are indeed overweight or obese. This means having a BMI (body mass index; see page 32) of 25 to 29.9 kg/m² if you're overweight or 30 kg/m² and up if you're obese. At a BMI of 30, a person is said to have stage 1 obesity. Stage 2, which carries a great deal more risk for diabetes as well as cancer and cardiovascular disease, begins at a BMI of 35. Stage 3 obesity, which used to be called "morbid obesity" as an indication of its severity, is defined as having a BMI of 40 or above. At each stage it gets harder to lose weight, and the risk of other illnesses, including cancer and cardiovascular disease, goes way up. With people at such an advanced state of obesity, bariatric surgery is sometimes recommended (to learn more about this option, see chapter 12).

As we discussed in chapter 2, BMI is a shorthand tool we use to estimate what percentage of your body weight is fat by dividing your weight in kilograms by your height in meters squared. It doesn't take into account your age, bone density, or muscle development. If you have very large bones or are an extremely well-toned athlete, a higher-than-normal BMI may be misleading. You may well be an appropriate weight for your build and musculature. While "normal" BMI ranges from 18.5 to 24.9 kg/m^2, if you are seventy or older, a BMI of 26 kg/m^2 may actually be the healthiest weight. But for most people, the standard ranges are helpful as a check. Having a BMI within healthy parameters correlates with the least risk for getting sick or dying prematurely.

THE PROBLEM WITH EXCESS FAT

Our muscle cells don't just enable us to move; they also have a metabolism to burn fuel and keep us lean and active. Conversely, our fat cells are not just inert storage cells. In recent years we've learned that they contain estrogen receptors, a hormone whose excess is associated with a number of cancers. Indeed, several cancers, such as breast, colorectal, and pancreatic, are clearly associated with fat. A woman who is obese (BMI over 30) has a 33 percent greater risk of breast cancer than a woman of normal weight. Increased risk of thyroid cancer, endometrial cancer, ovarian cancer, kidney cancer, pancreatic cancer, and cancer of the gallbladder are also associated with obesity. So are many chronic medical problems, such as high blood pressure, heart disease, stroke, sleep apnea, osteoarthritis, acid reflux, and gout, especially in men.

Fat cells also produce toxic chemicals—cytokines—that cause inflammation and may play a role in insulin resistance. And more and more, we're realizing that diabetes is an inflammatory disease. That's why our dietary program, The Blood Sugar Budget (see chapter 8), not only lowers blood sugar but also relieves inflammation and boosts nutrition to encourage weight loss.

This normal BMI range is helpful to know because judging your proper body weight by looking around at the mall, in the supermarket aisles, or at the local pizza parlor can be misleading. Remember that 70 percent of the population is overweight or obese. That means that, on average, at least seven out of ten people you see in your daily life are carrying around too much fat and have a shape that should not be considered the ideal. We've lost perspective on what is normal. Glance at a group photo of the public from the 1950s or 1960s. Everyone looks so skinny. But that's how human beings are supposed to look. Two decades ago, people were in many ways healthier than they are now. They were more physically active, they ate smaller portions, and the balance of fats, proteins, and carbohydrates in their diet was very different from what it is today.

When we speak about a normal weight, we're not talking about cosmetic appearances here; we're speaking of health. Despite a brief flurry of talk about "healthy obesity," which argued that heavy people were actually less susceptible to disease—a theory quickly proven untrue—mortality numbers don't lie. Being overweight or obese leads to greatly increased risk of prediabetes and diabetes as well as a host of other chronic diseases such as heart disease and cancer.

METABOLIC SYNDROME

Some overweight and obese individuals have a condition called "metabolic syndrome," which is a big risk factor for diabetes. Many people with metabolic syndrome are prediabetic, but not all. Prediabetes and metabolic syndrome create a perfect storm that frequently results in type 2 diabetes. Although there is no one clinical test for metabolic syndrome, it's fairly easy for doctors and nutritionists to spot. A hallmark symptom is abdominal, or central, obesity, which means excess fat around the middle—what we call an "apple-shaped body." In addition, to be diagnosed with metabolic syndrome, a person must have at least two of the following conditions:

- Elevated glucose level
- High blood pressure
- High triglycerides
- Low HDL (the so-called "good" cholesterol)

All these factors contribute to a much greater risk of developing diabetes, cardiovascular disease, and stroke. There are strong indications that internal fat around the midsection prevents insulin's message from ever reaching its target cells.

. . .

Whether you have metabolic syndrome or are simply overweight or obese, if you have minimally high blood sugar, it is a huge benefit to catch the disease at this preliminary stage. For one thing, with proper medical management and lifestyle changes, there is a good chance you can prevent prediabetes from progressing to type 2 diabetes, and in many cases, you may be able to actually *reverse* the disease so that you do not need lifelong medication. Even though there is a good likelihood that any elevated glucose has already caused some microvascular damage, it may well be minimal, and lowering your numbers now could allow you to escape damaging long-term complications in the future. I cannot emphasize too strongly: prediabetes is a call to arms. There are many conditions and health problems over which we have no control. Prediabetes, though, can be conquered with proper lifestyle modifications, which will benefit your mental and physical capabilities and improve your overall health in the process. But a diagnosis of prediabetes must be taken seriously right away.

DEALING WITH PREDIABETES

As I tell my patients, managing your prediabetes and hopefully reversing it is mostly about committing to a healthier lifestyle. It requires paying attention to your doctor's recommendations, taking any prescribed medications religiously, making better choices about what you eat and drink, and taking charge of your physical and emotional well-being. Regular exercise is a major component.

Halting and reversing prediabetes requires:

- Managing your medications
- Making dietary changes
- Losing weight
- Being physically active
- Reducing stress
- Getting enough sleep

Manage Your Medications

No one wants to take another pill. Maybe you're suspicious of the expense or side effects of pharmaceuticals. Or maybe you view the need to take a prescription as a weakness or personal failure. (If you believe that your lab results are borderline and imagine dropping ten pounds and whipping yourself into shape in a couple of months, you could be reluctant to admit what is perceived as the defeat of accepting a prescription from your doctor.) Yet halting the rise in blood sugar and, in fact, reversing it down to a normal or near-normal level as soon as possible is vital for preventing the damaging side effects of elevated blood glucose.

To cure prediabetes so that you don't need medication for life, a prescription is often beneficial in the short run. Lowering blood sugar is critical. Until you are confident that you can bring it under control naturally, it's essential that you work closely with your doctor or other health care practitioners to monitor your progress and take whatever medications are necessary on a daily basis without fail.

We used to give patients six months to a year to lose weight and adjust their lifestyle before we prescribed any drugs. But the best intentions have a way of stretching out from weeks to months, before petering out to daydreams in which we imagine what we'll do when we're ready. Sometimes "now" simply feels too stressful. We plan to make all those good changes after the baby is born, after the child is married, after you get a new job, after your next birthday, when your nerves calm down, when your boss goes on vacation. But more recently we've learned that elevated glucose of any sort damages tiny blood vessels in the peripheral nerves, retina, kidneys, and elsewhere much sooner than we'd imagined, and the excess sugar circulating in our bodies contributes to so-called hardening and obstruction of the arteries at a very early stage. So now I usually give motivated patients two to three months before handing them a prescription and recommending a nutritionist. These days a good nutritionist recommends appropriate physical activity as well as dietary plans. If you have no impulse to lose weight or exercise, I would recommend you take a single drug, usually metformin, immediately. If the lifestyle changes are successful and your counts go down sufficiently, then I would wean you from the drugs. But our priorities as doctors have definitely changed: first get that blood sugar down, then focus on keeping it down naturally so that the pharmaceuticals can be dispensed with.

NATURAL SUPPLEMENTS

In addition to pharmaceutical medicines, which you'll learn about in chapter 5, there are several natural supplements that may be helpful in the control and improvement of prediabetes. By "natural," we mean the substance is derived from a plant or is a vitamin or mineral. It is very important to keep in mind, though, that these need to be taken in therapeutic doses—doses that have an effect on the body. Consequently, they can have side effects, albeit much more minor than those of most pharmaceutical drugs, and they can interact with other medications you may be taking. So even though these substances can be purchased without a prescription and are available in your local drugstore or health food store, or on the Internet, it is imperative that you run it by your doctor, registered dietitian nutritionist, or pharmacist to make sure there will be no harmful interactions. That said, here a few a natural supplements that may be helpful:

Curcumin extract: A nine-month controlled trial suggested that curcumin extract, which is derived from the spice turmeric, in therapeutic doses of 750 mg twice a day with meals, improved the vigor of beta cells and prevented progression of prediabetes to type 2 diabetes over a three-year period. Other studies have suggested that this supplement may reduce activity of the toxic cytokines present in fat cells. Except for possible gastrointestinal irritation in a few individuals, this supplement appears to be quite safe. But even though it can be obtained over the counter, it's best to check with your physician or pharmacist to make sure it won't interact with any other medications you are taking.

Chromium picolinate: A number of studies have suggested that chromium picolinate enhances insulin sensitivity. It is often prescribed to women who have type 2 diabetes as a result of polycystic ovarian syndrome (PCOS). Chromium is a mineral common in many foods, but it can be deficient in a diet high in processed foods. As with any supplement, discuss this with your doctor or nutritionist before you take it. Despite many claims in the popular media, chromium picolinate has not been proven effective as a weight loss drug.

Alpha lipoic acid (ALA): Alpha lipoic acid is a powerful natural antioxidant, one that is vital in expediting the chemical reactions that allow a cell to produce energy. In appropriate amounts, it has been shown to improve glycemic control in patients with type 2 diabetes, but because it may lower blood sugar, you should alert your doctor if you are taking ALA, especially if you are prescribed metformin or another diabetes medication, to make sure you are not at risk for hypoglycemia. Reactions to ALA vary; some people report gastrointestinal symptoms.

Vitamin D: Although not a smoking gun to prove cause and effect, we do know that people with robust to normal vitamin D levels are less likely to have type 2 diabetes. Because vitamin D has been associated with other health benefits and is essential in maintaining bone health, it makes sense to make sure you're getting enough. A simple blood test will determine your serum vitamin D levels. Current government regulations say 30 ng/ml is the minimum normal, but many practitioners feel this number is too low. Some doctors and nutritionists aim for 50 to 60; I am happy if my patients are up to 40 or 50. If a blood test is not practical for you, it is safe to take 1,000 IU a day unless you have liver or kidney damage. Make sure what you buy is vitamin D_3 and not vitamin D_2, which is a less active form. And because it is fat soluble, be sure to take it with breakfast or another meal that includes a little fat.

Psyllium: Psyllium is a natural source of both soluble and insoluble fibers. Together, these fibers add bulk, help stools bind together, aid in preventing reabsorption of cholesterol, and modulate the digestion of carbohydrates, which can keep blood sugar on a more even keel. I'd rather you get your fiber from your diet, but if you don't, psyllium can help until you start to do the heavy lifting in your nutrition program.

Make Dietary Changes

Some people—especially Hispanics from Puerto Rico or Native Americans from the southwestern United States, as well as people of African American ancestry—have a significantly increased propensity toward high blood sugar. Some of the causes are cultural, but they can also be environmental or genetic.

For example, when Native Americans were forced off their land and herded onto reservations where there was no means of support, the government supplied them with rations such as white flour and lard. Did you know that fried bread, an incredibly unhealthy food that many consider to be a traditional Native American staple, arose only by necessity in the late 1880s? It is not a traditional food, though by now it is indigenous to the culture and probably one of the least healthy foods you could eat in terms of diabetes and obesity. Many poorer ethnic groups also live in communities that don't have good food stores or supermarkets. We call these places "food deserts" because it is so hard to find decent fresh produce and other healthy foods. But many people live in neighborhoods where vegetables and fruits are plentiful, and it comes down to the choices they make when buying food. A bag of chips or an apple—which would you choose? There seems to be a genetic component as well, especially for very slim people who cannot control their blood sugar levels.

But no matter what your risk or genetic profile, making the wrong choices about what to eat pushes glucose levels ever higher. First of all, excess calories of any kind are detrimental. If you take in more energy than you need, you're going to convert that energy into fat—which, as we've learned, simply feeds the blood sugar spiral. Modifying your diet to the appropriate number of calories for your height, age, and activity level is essential. Your doctor or a nutritionist who is a registered dietitian can best calculate the right diet for you, which almost always involves portion control as well as selecting the right foods. In addition to *how much* you eat, you need to take a very close look at *what* you eat. Our Blood Sugar Budget (see chapter 8) will start you out with the right framework for what you should eat. Going forward, a nutritionist can further tailor the program to your individual needs and food preferences.

Lose Weight

If your doctor has told you that you need to lose weight, begin by losing at least 5 to 7 percent of your weight and keeping it off for four months or longer. Once you start to lose weight, your blood pressure goes down, and you establish a regular routine of physical activity, then you can speak to your doctor about trying to wean yourself from your medication. Do not simply stop taking your pills on your own. You need to understand how to monitor yourself; it may be that you need to keep taking a smaller dose for a while, or you may be ready to go it alone.

What is exciting about managing prediabetes is that you are in charge. It's the decisions *you* make that will determine whether you progress to type 2 diabetes or return to a normal state in which your body uses insulin properly and your fasting plasma blood sugar remains below 100 mg/dl. Another benefit is that any of the changes you make to improve your blood sugar status will also improve your overall well-being, your energy level, how you look and feel, and how you think.

Whether you are round in the middle like an apple or just carry excess fat all over, the first order of business for anyone who wants to control or reverse prediabetes is weight loss. Losing even just 5 to 7 percent of your current body weight can make a huge difference in your health. If you're 220 pounds, that means losing 11 to 15 pounds. Although weight loss is almost always challenging, that's a lot easier than the ideal goal you might set for a bikini body with a weight loss of 50 to 75 pounds. Setting unrealistic goals is counterproductive and discouraging

One easy way to lose weight is to set yourself up for success rather than failure. Tell yourself you need to lose three pounds first. Even with modest changes to your diet, you could probably do that in two weeks at most. Then just repeat the program until you reach your goal. When you've lost enough to lower your glucose, reduce your blood pressure, and perhaps even improve your cholesterol numbers, then you can set about establishing a new goalpost.

Working with a registered dietitian nutritionist to establish a proper diet that works for you is an investment that will pay for itself. For one thing, there is no one "diabetes diet." Treatment for the disease must be individualized, and experts argue about which type of diet is best. Current evidence indicates that the same healthy diet that works for individuals who are disease free is equally appropriate for people with prediabetes or even type 2 diabetes.

But you are unique. What foods you prefer, what other medications you take, and what your lifestyle is like will affect your diet. Some people have individualized blood sugar responses to certain foods. So be alert to how you feel about what you eat. But you need to begin somewhere.

Our Blood Sugar Budget gives you a great place to start. Followed properly and paired with recommended physical activity, it will lower your blood sugar, help you lose weight, and reduce inflammation. With this program, you can make your own choices within a prescribed framework, and you'll learn the foods you *must* eat as well as those you should avoid.

If you need further help, or if you find you're still having unpleasant symptoms, we urge you to consult a registered dietitian nutritionist. It may be you have a hidden food allergy or intolerance, which a professional can identify. You may need more intensive counseling to help you achieve your goals. A nutritionist can also suggest supplements that might help improve your prediabetes, depending upon what other medications you are taking. Or you may have another underlying medical condition that needs to be treated by a physician.

A healthy diet involves a lot more than just giving up calories. Many people, especially women, torture themselves trying to lose weight on 1,200-calorie-per-day diets while eating nothing but refined carbohydrates. They are miserable, and they're starving themselves. Ironically, many people who are overweight or obese are actually what we call *undernourished*. They're getting more than enough calories and sometimes too much protein, but in terms of fiber, vitamins, and minerals as well as the essential fatty acids, they are sorely lacking. And this affects weight. Even if you are eating very few calories, if you're not getting the nutrients you need for good health, you are going to be much more likely to binge. Your metabolism may also be slowed, because we need fiber and certain vitamins and minerals to facilitate the metabolism of fats and carbohydrates in the gut. And likely you'll feel tired all the time.

Most people with diabetes or prediabetes have some idea of what they shouldn't eat, starting with sugar and refined white starches. But it's just as important to be knowledgeable about what you *should* eat: like enough leafy green vegetables, natural sources of calcium, and healthy fats like olive oil. That's where our Blood Sugar Budget comes in so handy. Sacrificing what's "bad" without adopting what's "good" won't get you where you need to be.

Most people with prediabetes or type 2 diabetes understand that added sugar is not good for them. If something tastes sweet, it will raise the blood glucose levels. (Excessive sugar also causes tooth decay, weakens bones, contributes to obesity, is a major risk factor for diabetes, and is even linked to some cancers.) Most patients also know (even without dietary counseling) that they should avoid candy, ice cream, cookies, pastries, and cakes except as treats. Unless you have a sugar addiction, the biggest problem comes from hidden sources of sugar.

White bread, white rice, potato chips, fried potatoes, mashed potatoes, crackers, and pasta are all powerful sources of carbohydrates that get quickly converted to sugar when you digest them. So even if you eat a sugar-free cookie made with artificial sweetener, you are loading up on carbs that have the same effect in the body as sugar itself. To paraphrase Shakespeare: a carbohydrate by any other name is just as dangerous.

Transforming your diet to a healthy one is not just a matter of knowing what you *shouldn't* eat, like refined carbohydrates, pasta, soda, and other sugar-sweetened beverages. It's knowing what you *should* eat—vegetables, fruits, whole grains, lean meats, nuts, olive oil—that will make such a big difference in your health and push back that prediabetes.

Be Physically Active

But diet alone is not enough. Physical activity has been proven even more effective than diet in terms of improving overall health and cardiovascular well-being. The rule of thumb is thirty to forty-five minutes of moderate exercise *every day*. Walking is excellent exercise, and you can break it up, doing ten or fifteen minutes at a clip. Take the stairs if possible, park your car in the farthest part of the lot, walk around the mall in bad weather, or take your dog out. If you have a lot of leg and knee pain because you are heavy, walking may be difficult or impossible. Okay, so look around at what you can do. Most senior citizen centers and YMCAs have exercise programs customized for people who are physically impaired. You could do chair exercises or water aerobics, or perhaps tai chi, which helps improve flexibility and balance. Anything physical you do improves your cardiovascular health and can help lower blood sugar.

Reduce Stress

Constantly feeling stressed maintains high levels of cortisol, a hormone we need if we are in danger and need a burst of energy to escape a predator. To fulfill its function, which was intended for emergencies, cortisol stimulates the liver to produce glucose for extra energy. But if cortisol is pumping out all the time, it suppresses the immune system, retards bone formation and breakdown of fat, increases insulin resistance, and leads to higher blood sugar levels.

Day to day, you may or may not be aware of how stressed you are. Big aggravations, like being tied up in traffic, getting chewed out by your boss, or worrying about bills at the end of the month may be obvious nail-biters. But loneliness, depression, or disappointment in a relationship or enterprise can provide background stress that affects you every minute of the day though you may not be aware of it.

The best way to relieve stress is to remove the thing that is upsetting you, which may or may not be possible. If money is a problem, for example, you can cut down on luxuries and entertainment, but that mortgage or rent is still due every month. Being proactive will help, but it may not be enough. If stress remains in your life, as it does in most people's—mine included—you need to learn ways to alleviate the physical expression of that stress.

Exercise is a great stress reliever, emotionally as well as physically. Because stress is a cycle—you feel it emotionally, then you react physically, which reinforces the emotion, which heightens the stress you feel—you can attack the problem either way. Relaxing physically or calming yourself emotionally will help, and the two together are dynamite.

The best form of exercise is the one you will actually do. Your choices are all over the place. Just choose something that is not unduly demanding, too expensive, or boring to you. For psychological relief there is also a range of options, from meditation or yoga to spiritual or psychological counseling to spending more time playing with your children, grandchildren, or a pet. Rewarding yourself for helping yourself is also a good strategy, whether you buy yourself a small gift or treat yourself to a manicure.

Get Enough Sleep

We often think of sleep just in terms of rest, but in fact, we've learned that an awful lot goes on while we're snoozing. The body does a lot of internal housekeeping and resetting of hormones. When not enough time is allowed for these processes to take place, metabolism can slow down. Surprising as it may seem, not getting enough sleep—at least seven and preferably eight hours—is associated with weight gain and obesity.

A more direct way lack of sleep affects weight is in terms of added calories. If we stay up long enough after supper, we get hungry again. After five or six hours of wakefulness after dinner, who doesn't crave a midnight snack? An extra 250 calories or more for half a sandwich and a glass of milk or a bowl of ice cream every night will add on half a pound a week.

Most of us don't have a lot of leeway in terms of when we can get up in the morning. There is work or a baby or a dog, and except on weekends, the time is probably the same every day. But we do have control over when we go to bed. So turn down the heat, turn out the lights, and turn off the TV and computer if you are serious about sleep.

. . .

And one other thing: if you smoke, do whatever you have to do to stop. Smoking has been definitively linked not only to lung cancer and COPD (chronic obstructive pulmonary disease) but also to heart disease and to type 2 diabetes. Programs to help you quit range from behavioral modification counseling to hypnosis, group therapy, and nicotine patches. Talk to your primary care provider to decide which is best for you and what is available in your geographic area.

We hope you found this chapter as informative and upbeat as we intended it to be. The good news about prediabetes is that it is manageable and in many cases even reversible. What's even better is that lifestyle modifications—especially diet and physical activity—can be more potent than pharmaceuticals; this allows you to take charge of your health naturally. And if your doctor prescribes one of the medications you'll read about in chapter 5, you'll see how the two together are extremely effective.

One challenge is that screening for elevated blood sugar does not always take place regularly, and the diagnosis is not always reported to the patient. So you have to be your own advocate for monitoring your blood sugar, knowing when it is too high, and understanding what you can do for yourself to lower it. Number one is losing weight, which goes hand in hand with better nutrition, both of which are addressed in our Blood Sugar Budget (see chapter 8). Number two is getting up off the couch or out of the car and moving. Reducing stress, getting enough sleep, and quitting smoking or heavy alcohol use, if necessary, will also help. And, of course, faithfully taking any medications your doctor prescribes is a given, along with any natural supplements you may want to try.

Sounds simple, doesn't it? But it adds up to a lot. And because any change is hard for all of us, you need and deserve help and encouragement. Regular counseling is the best way to guarantee success. So it's essential to partner with your doctor and find a registered dietitian nutritionist or diabetes educator who can keep you on track and help you over the hurdles. But you know what they say about silver linings, and there is definitely one here. If you are diagnosed with prediabetes and you rise to the challenge, it is very likely your health and vitality will become better than ever before—and your risk of a number of future chronic diseases will be greatly diminished.

CHAPTER 4

COMPLICATIONS FROM DIABETES

I HAVE A FRIEND who transformed a small company into a multimillion-dollar corporation. He has succeeded not just because of his strong work ethic, but also because he is observant and objective about his business decisions. Whenever he gets upset during a negotiation, he doesn't let it show or let his emotions cloud his judgment. My friend, however, is not as objective or diligent about his health. I am not his physician, but in the past he has hinted that he might have the "beginnings" of clogged arteries and "perhaps" diabetes. Recently, he had to be rushed to the hospital due to a massive infection that had overtaken his body. In the course of routine tests during that hospitalization, his doctors found that a very important artery of his heart was almost completely clogged. And when I visited him in the hospital, his doctor mentioned that my friend had not been taking care of his diabetes!

If my friend had paid as much attention to his health as he had done with his business, he would have known that his diabetes, if not treated aggressively, could contribute to heart disease, kidney disease, and even a compromised immune system. Luckily he survived his near-death experience and is now focusing much more on his health. You should, too, and here's why.

One of the frustrations of type 2 diabetes is not just the disease itself, but also all the complications that can occur over time. As blood overly saturated with sugar pumps through all the arteries and tiny blood vessels of the body every second of every day, damage occurs in almost every organ. That's why it's essential to get blood sugar under control as soon as possible, even if it means using insulin.

We don't fully understand the role of diabetes in vascular damage, but one premise that has been illustrated in animals explains that excess glucose ultimately inhibits the production of *nitric oxide*, a gas produced by the body that allows blood vessels to relax and expand. (Exercise, by the way, increases the production of nitric oxide.) Hyperglycemia keeps blood vessels tightly constricted.

When the arteries are constricted, they cannot accommodate the extra force that comes with exercise or certain stimulants like coffee. Instead, the blood in those arteries is under higher pressure—much like a pressure cooker. So with cramped space and a great deal of circulating sugar, damage easily occurs, especially in the tiny microscopic vessels that feed the nerves, eyes, and kidneys. That's why long-term uncontrolled diabetes can wreak such havoc, including greater risk of heart attack and stroke; wounds that won't heal, leading to amputation; and kidney damage, leading to dialysis. Not to mention an increased risk of Alzheimer's disease and other forms of dementia.

SHORT-TERM COMPLICATIONS

In order to reduce the risk of complications or reduce their impact as much as possible, it helps to know what they are, why they occur, and what you can do about them.

Hyperglycemia

Hyperglycemia, by definition, is a level of sugar in the blood above the accepted normal range. As I have mentioned repeatedly, elevated blood sugar in and of itself causes tissue damage, but having a blood sugar level that is extremely elevated can cause life-threatening changes in the body within a matter of hours. An extremely high blood sugar (and I am talking at least 300 mg/dl—remember, normal is under 100) can cause an imbalance in the delicate acid-base structure in the tissues of the body.

When the body can no longer use sugar as a source of energy, it starts breaking down fat and protein. One of the by-products of these two alternative sources of energy is *ketones.* A high level of circulating ketones not only damages tissues, but can also cause confusion, unconsciousness, and eventually coma. Excessively high ketones, a condition also called "metabolic ketoacidosis," usually occurs with type 1 diabetes, but it can affect those with type 2 as well if their blood sugar is wildly out of control.

Basically, there are three modes of treatment for hyperglycemia. Because the goal is to lower blood sugar and keep it controlled as quickly as possible, if your blood sugar does not go down, or if it goes up, treatment has to be maximized. Don't take it as a sign of failure if your doctor ups your regimen. It may well be through no fault of your own that increased medication is needed. Insulin used to be the drug of last resort. Now many physicians are turning to it sooner to lower elevated blood sugar in order to prevent the awful complications detailed in this chapter.

Here are the three methods your doctor will recommend to treat your hyperglycemia:

1. Diet and exercise
2. Oral drugs
3. Injected insulin

Remember, insulin is not the enemy: a *lack* of insulin is. If you are eating improperly or not being physically active, well, then you know what you have to do. You have to step up your game! Once the medications are working well, when you feel your diet and exercise are under control and you've lost enough weight, your doctor can try weaning you off one or more of your medications.

Hypoglycemia

This is when the sugar in your blood drops too low. Actually, I consider hypoglycemia to often be more dangerous than hyperglycemia. Its symptoms come upon you more quickly, and the dangers associated with hypoglycemia are very obvious. Remember, glucose is the brain's favorite food. Hypoglycemia is dangerous because if left unchecked, it can lead to unconsciousness and even seizures.

Because reining in blood sugar to lower and lower numbers has been shown to be significantly beneficial for preventing damage to blood vessels, doctors are treating type 2 diabetes more aggressively at an earlier stage. Goals for optimum blood sugar for diabetics used to be higher than for so-called healthy individuals. In other words, we used to let patients with diabetes slide, allowing them to live with blood sugars that were a bit above normal. Not anymore. Now we see the blood sugar goals of diabetics and nondiabetics coming closer and closer together.

If you are being treated for diabetes and taking drugs to lower your blood sugar, you should be alert for any signs of hypoglycemia. Symptoms of low blood sugar may include one of more of the following:

- Excessive weakness and fatigue
- Cold, clammy skin
- Increased heart rate
- Dizziness
- Blurred vision
- Extreme hunger
- Nausea
- Headache
- Unusual irritability
- Confusion
- Night sweats and nightmares
- Inappropriate sweating
- Rapid heart rate

Your body is vigilant, and it can overcorrect. It is not medication alone that can cause hypoglycemia. Blood sugar is also affected by stress and illness as well as diet and exercise. There are many times, even given constant medication, when you may be at risk for your blood sugar level becoming too low. It may be due to that parking ticket, those extra ten minutes on the treadmill, or skipping breakfast because you woke up late.

As a remedy for hypoglycemia, I recommend that you always carry glucose tablets or gels with you. These come in a choice of fruit flavors, and they are easy to stash in a pocket or purse. Each tablet contains 15 grams of easily absorbed carbohydrate—usually pure glucose. Two would be roughly equivalent to the amount of carbohydrate you'd get from a slice of bread. These tablets are better, though, because they are glucose in its pure state.

Therefore, it enters the bloodstream much more rapidly because it doesn't require digestion. Taken one at a time at fifteen-minute intervals, anywhere from one to three will probably stabilize you. Take another only if you still feel shaky. You need pure glucose only when you are really trembling or dizzy; that is, at the point of passing out. Don't overdo it, or you'll raise your blood sugar too high. Follow up with a blood sugar check, if you can.

More often, if you are aware of the symptoms of hypoglycemia, you can prevent it from occurring in the first place by eating sensibly. If you feel a drop, without going into the more severe symptoms just described, you can bring your levels back up with a nutritious snack. It's a good idea to acquaint yourself with these symptoms and be sensitive to them, so you don't reach the point where you need instant relief. Illness such as trauma or a fever can make blood sugar go up, in which case it is liable to fall. Also, strenuous exercise—including, if you're lucky, strenuous sex—can cause a spike.

Try to anticipate your activity level and adjust your carbohydrates ahead of time. (If you are taking short-acting insulin, you should discuss with your physician the possibility of lowering your dose by a unit or two if you know you will be exercising strenuously for two hours or longer. Have your doctor or diabetes educator instruct you on how to calculate how much of an adjustment to make.)

If you feel a drop after a strenuous workout, consume a measured amount of carbohydrate to bring you back up. If you're not about to pass out, it's an even better idea to pair that carbohydrate with some fat and/or protein to maintain blood sugar levels over time. Good choices are:

- Small glass (4 ounces) fruit juice or a few pieces of dried fruit for immediate response
- A 6-ounce (⅔ cup) glass of skim or 1 percent milk (surprise—even low-fat dairy is loaded with sugar!)
- Half an apple or pear and a small slice of good cheese
- Half a peanut-butter-and-jelly sandwich on whole grain bread
- Half a snack pack of raisins with a tablespoon of nuts

Following our Blood Sugar Budget (see chapter 8) helps avoid hypoglycemia because you are eating smaller meals at regular intervals, with healthy snacks in between, which will keep your blood sugar on an even keel.

LONG-TERM COMPLICATIONS OF TYPE 2 DIABETES

As we've said, it's the damage to the tiny blood vessels throughout the body over time that makes type 2 diabetes such a potent silent killer. It's always difficult to discuss these possible complications with a patient, because they are scary and depressing. But this knowledge is an important part of your self-management of the disease, because knowing what can happen allows you to take all the steps you can to prevent or alleviate these consequences. And take heart, because losing weight, eating a nutritious diet, maintaining a regular program of physical activity, and reducing stress as much as possible will all help you sidestep the devastation of long-term hyperglycemia.

On the other hand, if you think that just because you can't feel it, nothing is happening, maybe this discussion will be a wake-up call. If you think you can take your pills or leave them, or if you think your medication is a substitute for eating well and exercising, you may be in for a shock. Any of these complications could happen to you.

Blindness

Loss of vision caused by retinopathy, or damage to the retina, is one of the first complications that can occur due to elevated blood sugar. Blurred vision is sometimes one of the first symptoms of undiagnosed type 2 diabetes. Here's why: the retina lies at the back of the eye, with the optic nerve at its center. It is laced with an incredibly complex network of smaller nerves and nourished by an intricate web of blood vessels and tiny capillaries. When elevated blood sugar damages some of these small blood vessels, the eye tries to compensate by growing more of them, often erratically, and in a way that is detrimental to vision. Over time, vision is distorted and blindness eventually occurs.

To manage your eye health, lower your blood sugar as soon as possible and keep it down:

- If you are overweight or obese, lose at least 5 to 7 percent of your current body weight.
- Eat a nutritious diet, with special attention to getting enough vitamins A, D, and E; lutein and zeaxanthin (both found in green leafy vegetables); and copper, zinc, and omega-3s—all are especially

important for eye health. A consultation with a registered dietitian nutritionist to evaluate your diet and prescribe any necessary supplements is highly advised, because when it comes to supplements, more is not better. It is always best to get these nutrients first from your food.

- Maintain a regular physical activity program of at least thirty minutes every day (again, this does not have to be all at once).

- Take any medications your doctor has prescribed without fail. Every other day won't do it.

- Make sure you have an eye examination with an ophthalmologist—not just an optometrist—at diagnosis and then once a year. An ophthalmologist is a medical doctor who can give your eyes a thorough examination, checking for glaucoma, cataracts, and macular degeneration in addition to retinal vascular damage. Go back sooner if you notice any change in your vision. New laser surgery techniques can control some of the damage from uncontrolled vascular growth in the eye. Make sure you don't miss the appointment: have your ophthalmologist send you a reminder. If you move, make sure you update your address. Also, keep a list of doctors and yearly appointments in a written book or on your smart phone or computer with a calendar reminder.

Kidney Failure

As your blood passes through the kidneys, which contain a vast network of tiny blood vessels, proteins and minerals are filtered to maintain your body's sodium and potassium balance and balance your blood pressure. Essentially, this filtering controls the vital electrolytes in your blood. These tiny vessels are delicate and easily damaged by elevated glucose. An early sign of diabetes is excessive urination as your body tries to eliminate the excess sugar. In fact, the urine of people with very high blood sugar is sweet, which is how the formal name for the disease, *diabetes mellitus*—literally "sweet urine"— came about.

As the situation worsens, more and more proteins as well as glucose are lost in the urine. The first symptom of decreased kidney function is no symptom at all. As the kidneys start to fail, there is no pain; there is no decrease in urine production. In other words, you don't know that the kidneys have begun to fail. In the beginning of *nephropathy* ("sick kidneys"), the kidneys don't filter as well as they used to. Mind you, even with mild kidney insufficiency, the amount of work they do is still enough to clean out the toxins produced every day, but that work isn't as efficient as when they are completely healthy. Only certain blood tests will show this decrease in function.

As renal insufficiency worsens, some changes show up in your routine blood tests. Since the kidneys are able to filter less plasma every minute, the *creatinine level*, which measures a toxin related to protein metabolism, will increase and the *glomerular filtration rate* (GFR) will decrease. Someone in the early stages of kidney damage still will not even know this is happening, because she will feel nothing.

As the kidney's ability to filter diminishes, many of the proteins that would have otherwise been retained in the blood will "leak" out through the kidneys and into the urine. One of the main proteins we look for is called *albumin.* Therefore, a simple urine analysis might reveal protein in the urine.

When the kidneys are irreparably damaged and the toxins build up to a dangerous level, the only thing that can save you from certain death is external cleansing of the blood. This is called *dialysis.* Dialysis is a mechanized form of blood purification, which allows a machine to take over what the body cannot do. The patient's bloodstream is connected to a machine and then slowly filtered and returned to the body over a period of hours.

Obviously, the best medicine is to avoid kidney failure in the first place. Here's how to do it:

- Lower your blood sugar as soon as possible and keep it down.

- Control other health problems that could speed kidney damage, primarily high blood pressure. It's bad enough to have one disease that causes kidney damage. Who needs a double whammy?

- Have your urine checked for albumin and GFR at least on a yearly basis. GFR measures how much plasma your kidneys are able to filter every minute. When you go for your annual check-up and your doctor orders routine blood tests, a complete metabolic panel, including a GFR, is almost always part of the package. In a healthy adult, this number is above 60 ml/min. At 30 ml/min, there is moderate loss of effective kidney function. Total failure occurs around 15 ml/min. Obviously, we don't want it to ever get that low. So if your GFR is going down, it's important to have your doctor measure it more frequently—at least every six months, or more often if kidney damage is evident. If you do have reduced kidney function, your doctor can prescribe medications to help and a dietitian can outline a way of eating that takes some of the burden off the kidneys. If you do not respond positively to these medications, you should see a kidney specialist, called a *nephrologist*. Of course, this is all at the recommendation of your physician. So a close, candid relationship is essential.

- If you are overweight or obese, lose at least 5 to 7 percent of your current body weight.

- Eat a nutritious diet with special attention to reducing the sodium content of your food. Don't use added salt; try lemon juice and spices to perk up flavors. Avoid processed foods that are high in sodium, which you can tell from reading the label. Sodium content has to be listed by law. Don't use salt substitutes; they are just another form of sodium. In salt-sensitive individuals, salt boosts blood pressure. The DASH diet, which is similar to our Blood Sugar Budget but much lower in sodium, has been proven effective at lowering blood pressure naturally.

Note: African Americans are at increased risk for developing diabetes-related kidney problems. Therefore, you must pay extra attention to controlling hypertension and diabetes. As an aside, the GFR in African Americans is also higher than Caucasians, due to higher levels of lean muscle mass and creatinine production.

Heart Disease and Stroke

Cardiovascular disease resulting in heart attack or stroke is *the* leading cause of death in America, responsible for more than 600,000 deaths a year. But before I proceed, let's get some medical terms defined and cleared up. Many people use the terms *heart attack* or *stroke* interchangeably, but they are not the same thing at all.

Heart Attack (Myocardial Infarction): The heart is a muscle that has to pump in order for the rest of your body to get blood. Much like putting the oxygen mask on yourself before anyone else in case of an airplane emergency, the heart gives itself blood before it pumps blood to the rest of the body. It supplies itself with blood through its own arteries. Each artery is responsible for supplying blood to a specific section of the heart. If a heart artery clogs up, that portion of the heart will not receive blood and eventually die off. Much as a clogged-up sprinkler will cause a section of lawn to die, an artery that's congested with plaque made of fat and cholesterol will permanently cause a section of heart tissue to die when the blood supply can't get through. That is called a myocardial infarction (MI). Some people call this a *heart attack*, and others refer to the pain caused by an MI as a heart attack. For our purposes, both terms can be used interchangeably.

Stroke (Cerebral Vascular Accident, or CVA): The arteries that supply the brain with blood are for the most part very thin walled and fragile. Each of these arteries brings blood to a particular part of the brain. And each section of the brain has a special function: speech, hearing, arm movements, and so on. So if the artery that serves that area bursts or can no longer provide the area with blood, the area dies—and along with it, the function it was responsible for.

The rupture of a small artery in the brain can leave the victim unable to talk clearly or move one of his arms or legs. Such a rupture is technically called a *cerebral vascular accident*, or a *stroke*. The most likely cause of brain artery rupture is high blood pressure. Therefore, the most common cause of strokes is hypertension.

Stroke and heart attack have this in common: the continued normal function of the heart and the brain depends on the strength and health of the arteries that supply them with blood. Diabetes can weaken the arteries of both the brain and the heart. It can also lessen the amount of important substances like nitric oxide; this in turn can make the arteries more brittle and more likely to get clogged up or to burst.

To prevent heart attack and stroke:

- If you smoke, stop as soon as possible.
- Lower your blood sugar as soon as possible and keep it down.
- Lower your blood pressure to a normal range. This can be accomplished through diet, exercise, and/or medications.
- Lower your total cholesterol. This can be accomplished through diet, exercise, and/or medications.
- Decrease your LDL ("bad" cholesterol).
- Increase your HDL ("good" cholesterol).

- Take one baby aspirin (81 mg) per day.

- If you are overweight or obese, lose at least 5 to 7 percent of your current body weight.

- Eat a nutritious diet that avoids butter, red meat, and processed meats as much as possible. Get plenty of omega-3s. Eat fish at least three times a week: canned tuna, salmon, and sardines count. Choose "light" rather than "white" tuna for less possible exposure to mercury. And keep in mind that canned salmon and sardines with their bones are the most healthful because they are rich in calcium. Include as many vegetables as you can in your diet.

- Follow our Blood Sugar Budget (see chapter 8) for an appropriate nutritional balance. If you are an older adult, make sure you eat a little protein with every meal. We need a bit more as we age, and we have no storage facility for protein. Your body needs only a small amount of the essential amino acids, but if it doesn't get the protein it requires, it will take it from your muscles and organs.

- Enroll in a cardio-fitness class with a certified trainer. Make sure you've had a stress test or your doctor has otherwise approved your exercise program before you begin. If nothing else, make sure you walk a total of thirty to forty-five minutes a day every day of the week.

Neuropathy

One of the first outright symptoms of diabetes is *peripheral neuropathy*, which is usually manifested as a tingling in the fingers, hand, toes, legs, or feet. It occurs because the tiny blood vessels that nourish the nerves become damaged from excessive levels of glucose, and the nerves themselves begin to die. At first these symptoms may be minor annoyances that come and go. You may experience a coldness or numbness of the feet. It may last only a few hours. Perhaps in bed the pressure of the sheet on your toes becomes uncomfortable and a bit painful. All of these may be symptoms of early neuropathy.

If elevated blood sugar is left unchecked, over time the nerves cease to function. First you may experience pain, and eventually you may lose all sensation, especially on the soles of your feet. This is really danger-ous, because you won't feel cuts and blisters, which can develop serious infections. This can also affect balance, because if you can't feel the bottoms of your feet, the feet won't be able to send the necessary information to your brain to tense your knee tendons to stabilize your stance. This is why we sometimes fall over when we get up suddenly after a leg has "fallen asleep." But in real diabetic neuropathy, losing your balance may become a regular occurrence. You won't be able to walk well. Once mobility is gone, health goes into a downward spiral.

Another kind of nerve damage affects the autonomic, or unconscious, functioning of your body. Although it can extend to the heart and lungs, and even the sexual organs (see page 66), many years of uncontrolled diabetes and elevated blood sugar can especially impact the digestive system. Damage to nerves—especially to the vagus nerve, which controls stomach movement—can retard stomach emptying and cause slow motility of the gut. Technically called *gastroparesis*, this often leads to acid reflux and constipation. It can also lead to a decrease in appetite because of a sense of fullness. Two other kinds of neuropathy result in weakness in the trunk and pain in the legs and sudden weakness or pain almost anywhere in the body.

To prevent or manage neuropathy:

- Lower your blood sugar as soon as possible and keep it down.
- If you are overweight or obese, lose at least 5 to 7 percent of your current body weight.
- Eat a nutritious diet rich in vitamins and minerals.
- If you already have symptoms of gastroparesis, eat many small meals a day. Be sure to walk after each meal so that movement and gravity can assist in emptying your stomach.
- Consult with your physician or gastroenterologist about using certain medications that may induce the stomach to empty more quickly. Unfortunately, once the damage to the vagus nerve occurs, there is very little that can be done to repair it and restore natural function.

Nonhealing Infections

The main way for any sore to heal is to receive adequate blood flow. The blood contains everything that is necessary for healing: white blood cells, proteins, minerals, and so on. If blood does not reach a wound, there is no way that it will heal. Diabetes destroys blood vessels that carry oxygen and other nutrients to cells. Not only does diabetes destroy the main conduit for supplying blood, but it also weakens the immune system. There are a number of different kinds of sores, wounds, and infections that are more common with extended periods of elevated blood sugar.

For example, calcified sores that occur from eating too much phosphorus-rich food while undergoing dialysis (which is hard to avoid because there is phosphorus in almost all foods, especially in meats and dairy) are exceedingly painful and difficult to heal. They often result in critical infections.

FOOT CARE

Cuts, calluses, blisters, and sores on the feet pose a very real hazard for people with long-standing diabetes, especially if blood sugar has gone uncontrolled for long enough to cause neuropathy.

To care for your feet, follow these steps every day:

1. Keep your feet clean; wash them in warm water with mild soap. Check the water temperature with your hand before you dip your toe in, because if you have enough numbness, you could conceivably scald yourself.

2. Dry your feet thoroughly. Moisture, especially between the toes, provides a breeding ground for bacteria.

3. Purchase an angled, long-handled mirror. Telescoping mirrors designed specifically for diabetes foot inspection are sold in medical supply stores and on the Internet for less than $20. Inspect your feet carefully, checking between the toes, because you may have wounds you don't even feel. Look for cuts and sores and be suspicious of calluses and blisters, which can hide infected areas underneath.

4. To avoid cracks and chafing, moisturize your feet with a cream that contains bacteriostatic agents, such as Cetofil or Eucerin.

If you love your pedicures, make sure you go to only a quality salon with state-certified staff. Let them know you have diabetes, and caution them to be especially careful. Do not let anyone use a razor on you to shave off dead skin. A pumice stone is sufficient.

ERECTILE DYSFUNCTION AND DIABETES

It has been my experience as a physician that nothing makes a diabetic man want to control his blood sugar more then the realization that uncontrolled diabetes is one of the leading contributors to erectile dysfunction (ED). I wish it were a myth, but 35 to 75 percent of men who have diabetes are likely to get erectile dysfunction. This is two to three times greater than men who do not have diabetes. If you don't think that is significant, imagine making two to three times more money per year. It is a considerable difference! Research even suggests that erectile dysfunction may be an early indicator of diabetes, particularly in men aged forty-five and younger. Men with diabetes may experience the problem ten to fifteen years earlier than men without diabetes. The good news, however, is that there are ways to lessen the effect of diabetes on erectile dysfunction.

I strongly believe that in order for people to make a permanent improvement in their health they have to understand how things work and how a disease causes damage. We doctors call it the *pathophysiology* of a disease. This most certainly applies to diabetes and ED. Erectile dysfunction in particular has so many psychological connotations that it is often very embarrassing for a man who suffers from it to discuss with his physician. When you understand how the penis functions and how years of high blood sugar can permanently damage your ability to get and maintain an erection, you are more likely to see a physician and get that blood sugar under control, pronto!

When a man cannot get or maintain an erection, he often feels the condition is visual proof that he is somehow less of a man. This can also put a strain on a loving relationship. Society tends to believe that getting and maintaining an erection is a simple thing, but nothing could be further from the truth.

The Mechanics of an Erection

The penis is mostly made up of three spongy muscles: the *corpus spongiosum* and two side-by-side chambers called the *corpus cavernosum*. They are not really muscles, but sponge-like chambers into which blood flows. It is the pressure of the blood in those chambers that creates an erection. Imagine filling a long balloon with water. Anatomically, that is all an erection is. This may seem simple, but it is not.

The two *corpura cavernosa*, which are mainly responsible for the erection, are made of small arteries, veins, and empty chambers. Each small artery and vein is controlled by a smooth muscle fiber. What is unique about smooth muscle is that you cannot willfully control it. For example, you can flex your bicep at will because it is made of *striated muscle*. Striated muscle can be controlled by mental command. However, you cannot "think" your high blood pressure down, because arteries are made of smooth muscle. It takes an intricate cascade of nerves and chemicals to allow smooth muscle to function correctly.

When you have an erection, nerve signals from your brain or from the nerve endings in your penis cause the smooth muscle of the chambers to relax and the arteries to dilate. If you are aroused by something you see, hear, or smell, the stimulus will come from your brain. If you are aroused by your penis being touched, then the stimulation will come from the sacral nerve roots of your spinal cord. In either case, the end result is a rush of blood that fills the empty spaces of the corpus cavernosum and voilà, an erection! But again, the mechanics do not end here.

This blood that has just entered the corpus cavernosum needs to stay within the penis, or the erection will be lost almost immediately. The pressure of the blood in the chambers then causes a sheath of tissue around them to squeeze on the veins that normally allow blood to drain out of the penis. This pressure closes off the veins, trapping the blood within the penis and maintaining the rigidity of the erection. Once the excitement subsides, the nerves send different information to the smooth muscle. This now causes the sheath to relax, taking pressure off the veins and allowing blood to drain out of the penis, returning it to its flaccid state.

Those are just the mechanics visible to the naked eye. Even more complicated are the microscopic or tiny chemical events that must occur in order for an erection to happen. First and foremost, the penis must be stimulated neurologically in one of two ways: by touch or by the brain. In either case, the nerves need to be functioning correctly. We now know that after years of damage from elevated blood glucose, these nerves won't respond correctly. In one case, the nerves that connect to the brain do not receive the information correctly. In the second case, the nerves in the penis may already be a bit numb and not respond normally to stimulation. The result is the inability to have and maintain an erection.

Research shows that one of the main causes of ED in diabetics is damage to the *nitric oxide pathway*. As we've mentioned previously, nitric oxide is a chemical that is released into the bloodstream by the lining of the blood vessels. You could say that it acts as a messenger that tells the smooth muscles and arteries in the penis to relax and let the blood in. Studies have shown that elevated blood sugar damages the nitric oxide pathway. Therefore, elevated blood glucose leads to a decrease in nitric oxide, which leads to poorly relaxed arteries in the penis, which leads to decrease blood flow to the penis, which eventually causes erectile dysfunction.

Unfortunately, this is not the only illness linked to diabetes that contributes to ED. As you already know, diabetes is associated with both high blood pressure and high cholesterol—each of which separately contributes to erectile dysfunction. If you have either of these, or both, along with diabetes, your chance of having erectile dysfunction is even higher.

Constricted arteries cause hypertension, or high blood pressure. Constricted arteries also decrease blood flow. Some people call it poor circulation. Therefore, hypertension causes a decrease in blood flow throughout the whole body and prevents all of your organs from working efficiently. This includes the penis. You know what this means. High blood pressure leads to a decrease in blood flow to the penis, therefore making it more difficult, if not nearly impossible, to obtain a normal erection.

Diabetes is also associated with an increase in cholesterol; specifically, an increase in LDL, or "bad" cholesterol. LDL cholesterol can affect the ability of arteries to dilate, and increased LDL cholesterol results in fatty deposits, or plaques, in the arteries. Having elevated LDL cholesterol increases the likelihood that your arteries are partially plugged up, which decreases blood flow more than would occur with diabetes alone. This double whammy makes men with high cholesterol much more likely to have erectile dysfunction.

Besides these three proven associations between diabetes and erectile dysfunction, there are a few softer associations. (Pardon the pun!) Men who have diabetes are very often depressed at the state of their health. Depression can certainly contribute to a decrease in libido. Though ED is mainly caused by physical issues, the role of the mind is incredibly important. Remember, in order to get an erection you must first be relaxed.

Some men also respond to a diagnosis of diabetes by overdoing or restarting habits that are deleterious to getting an erection. The two main ones are drinking alcohol and cigarette smoking. Smoking in particular is a known contributor to erectile dysfunction. So not only does diabetes directly contribute to erectile dysfunction, but the denial that sometimes comes along with the diagnosis can also create behavior that only makes matters worse.

How to Treat Erectile Dysfunction

Now that we have discussed the potential causes of erectile dysfunction in a male diabetic, can anything be done to improve and normalize the situation? The answer is yes.

Normalize Your Blood Sugar: The first thing you must do is normalize your blood glucose. Research has shown this again and again. This book is chock-full of ways to do this, from diet to exercise to medications. It is crucial that you get your A1C down to the normal range. Though there is no guarantee that normalizing your A1C will make your erections normal again, without this happening there is very little chance of your erectile dysfunction improving.

There is some evidence that taking the amino acid L-arginine can increase the production of nitric oxide. Remember, it is the decrease in production of nitric oxide in diabetics that may contribute the most to ED. This supplement is not generally accepted as a therapy for diabetic erectile dysfunction, but L-arginine has minimal side effects and is benign enough that most men should give it a shot. Please consult your physician for further advice.

Normalize Your Blood Pressure: Weight loss and regular exercise can help you get your blood pressure back into the normal range. With a normal blood pressure you stand the best chance of normal erections. However, if diet and exercise alone don't improve your blood pressure, consult your physician for treatment with medications. Don't be embarrassed to tell your doctor about your ED, because *some*—though not all—blood pressure medications, especially beta blockers, can make erectile dysfunction worse. You want to make sure that the treatment doesn't worsen matters.

Normalize Your Cholesterol: The advice I offer here is very much the same as for hypertension. First try diet and exercise, but if after a few months your cholesterol does not decrease into the normal range, go see your physician and start on medication to reduce your cholesterol. It will decrease your chances of heart disease and probably improve your erectile dysfunction.

Normalize Your Life: Maintaining an ideal body weight and doing regular exercise will help in improving erectile dysfunction. It will also help with your body image, and that by itself may go a long way toward helping your ED.

Stop Smoking Cigarettes: Notice that we do not recommend you cut down on cigarette smoking. We suggest that you stop smoking completely, and there is no room for compromise on this one. Cigarettes alone are the number one contributor to poor blood flow to your extremities (of which the penis is one). Any man with erectile dysfunction who wants to strengthen his erections should not be smoking—at all. And smoking has recently been incontrovertibly linked to type 2 diabetes, as well—no excuses!

Accept and Conquer Your Diabetes: The depression and anxiety that sometimes come with being given a new diagnosis can certainly contribute to erectile dysfunction. By reading this book, you have committed to facing your diabetes head-on and conquering it. That is a great first step. Work with your health care professional closely and make him aware of any persistent sadness or changes in eating or sleeping patterns. These may all be signs of depression that may be contributing to your ED. Medications or sexual counseling may be the answer here.

Rule Out Other Causes: Get a good general physical examination to make sure you are otherwise healthy. Just because you have diabetes doesn't mean that you can't have other causes of erectile dysfunction. Ask your physician to check your testosterone level along with other hormones, including FSH, LH, prolactin, estradiol, and TSH. These will indicate whether there is a hormonal imbalance that may be playing a role in your ED. Your prostate must be working correctly in order to have a normal erection, and in some men an enlarged prostate (benign prostatic hypertrophy) may contribute to ED. Your physician should also check for vascular (circulation) and neurological causes of ED.

Consider Medications as Treatment: We have all heard about the little blue pill. There is a reason that Viagra is one of, if not the, best-selling medication in the United States, and for one reason: it works. This medication, along with its close relatives (Cialis, Levitra), is a phosphodiesterase type-5 inhibitor (PDE5). Quite simply, these normalize the chemicals that allow the blood vessels in the penis to dilate, thus improving the blood flow to the organ. These medications can work for hours or days, depending on the brand and dosage. Please consult your physician to see which one might be right for you.

If oral medications don't do the trick, then perhaps medications that are injected into the corpus cavernosum of the penis might be the best choice. Though the thought of injecting your penis to get an erection may be disturbing, these injections are almost always guaranteed to work. The needles are very small, and the results are almost immediate. Some examples are Alprostadil, Phetolamine, and Papavirine. Some intra-penile injections contain a mixture of all three. Recently these medications have been formulated into a cream that can be squirted into the urethra of the penis. Consult your physician about these options, too.

Consider Using Other Helpful Devices: There are a number of devices sold online or at adult stores that can help you achieve or maintain an erection. For instance, a penis ring that is placed at the base of the penis during sex will keep the blood within the penis. Another option is a vacuum device that can be used right before sex. It is placed on the penis and causes blood to be sucked into the penis. If these options fail to help, there are implants that can be surgically placed in the penis. Some are semi-rigid and malleable. Others are fully inflatable at the time needed. Once considered the only solution for men with ED, these devices have now been relegated to last-resort status.

It Happens to All of Us

Man to man, I can tell you that erectile dysfunction happens to all of us at one time or another. It is nothing to be ashamed of or embarrassed about. What would be a shame is if you let it go untreated, especially because there are so many excellent treatment options. What I want you to realize most of all, however, is that this is one more reason to take your diabetes very seriously and to conquer it. I commend you for reading this and getting informed. I am sure that this is the first step toward conquering your or your mate's erectile dysfunction.

ALZHEIMER'S DISEASE AND OTHER FORMS OF DEMENTIA

Many complications from diabetes contribute to Alzheimer's disease and other forms of dementia and at an earlier age than the more typical onset in previously healthy individuals. Loss of blood flow to the brain, inability to absorb nutrients, and the death of nerve cells all account for the fact that diabetes is associated with both vascular dementia and Alzheimer's disease. These are devastating conditions for both patient and family. What starts out as casual memory loss deteriorates into personality changes, profound memory loss, and eventual death.

Both insulin resistance and elevated blood sugar increase the risk of heart attack and stroke, which can damage blood vessels in the brain. As I've said before, glucose is your brain's favorite food. If its cells cannot receive the sugar from the blood, the brain will be deprived of energy, which can cause cell damage. The cellular inflammation caused by elevated blood sugar may also damage the brain. So can too much insulin, a powerful hormone that triggers many other hormonal and chemical reactions.

To prevent or manage Alzheimer's and other dementia:

- Lower your blood sugar as soon as possible and keep it down.

- If you smoke, quit immediately.

- If you are overweight or obese, lose at least 5 to 7 percent of your current body weight.

- Be vigilant about exercising. Strive for moderate exercise five days a week and vigorous exercise two days a week. The duration should be thirty to forty-five minutes. Many studies have associated ongoing, regular physical activity with improved cognitive function and memory. Exercise even trumps diet for proven effectiveness.

- Eat a nutritious diet. This is extremely important for cognitive, mental, and emotional health, especially as we age. Get enough B_6 and folate; B_{12} is also very important. Your doctor can test for these levels in your blood. It's easy to get enough B_6 and folate from your diet; it is contained in vegetables and whole grains. But as we age, our ability to absorb B_{12}, which is present in eggs, meat, fish, and dairy, may diminish. So even with a nutritious diet, some individuals may need B_{12} supplementation. Also, proton pump inhibitors, which so many people take for acid reflux, interfere with the absorption of B_{12}, as do certain gastrointestinal diseases. It's also important to obtain the right amount of folate, or folic acid, as its artificial form is called; taking in too much folic acid or B_6 over time can actually do permanent neurological damage. That's why it's important to work with your physician and a nutritionist to make sure you are getting what you need and not an excessive amount. A pregnant woman needs 800 mg of folate from all sources. Everyone else is fine with 400 mg per day, which can easily be provided by your diet if you follow our Blood Sugar Budget (see chapter 8).

- Remain social and engaged. Travel, if possible, and learn new things or give your brain a workout. Mental stimulation, social interaction, and learning new things are all associated with better cognitive function. Brain aerobics are essential!

THE TAKE-AWAY MESSAGE

As you can see, every single one of these complications caused by uncontrolled type 2 diabetes responds to three things:

- Weight loss
- An appropriate and nutritious diet
- Exercise and physical activity

In fact, in a landmark study called the Diabetes Prevention Program (DPP), researchers divided people at high risk for type 2 diabetes into two groups: one group was given diet and exercise programs; the second group was prescribed metformin (see page 80). The researchers wanted to see whether lifestyle changes could come close to the efficacy of a prescription medication. What they found was a surprise. Lifestyle changes, which were accompanied by intensive support and coaching, reduced the incidence of progression to type 2 diabetes by 58 percent compared to a control group. Metformin alone reduced the risk by only 31 percent compared to subjects given a placebo. For people with prediabetes, diet, exercise, and other lifestyle changes made a *bigger* difference than medication. This means that upon diagnosis, in addition to working with your doctor on your testing and pharmaceutical program, you should:

1. Begin by losing 5 to 7 percent of your body weight. Then, continue to lose weight at a modest pace—1 to 2 pounds a week at most—to achieve and maintain a healthy body weight for your age and sex.

2. Consult with a registered dietitian nutritionist to come up with a customized diet that lowers your blood sugar while taking into account any medications you are taking, your activity level, and any other medical conditions you may have. Studies have proven this extra support and counseling results in lower blood sugar and better outcomes in the long run.

3. Outline a program of ongoing movement and weight-bearing exercise that works for your lifestyle and physical abilities (see chapter 10 for some ideas).

An ounce of prevention is worth much more than a pound of cure. The reason we lay out these complications so graphically is to create awareness that even if the elevated blood sugar doesn't hurt, its long-term consequences are well worth avoiding. The good news is that a major recent study documented how effective our medical treatment and diabetes self-management techniques have been at reducing the number and severity of these complications.

CHAPTER 5

UNDERSTANDING MEDICATIONS THAT TREAT DIABETES

W E ARE SO LUCKY to be living in an age in which science has not only proven what causes many diseases but also has figured out ways to treat them by understanding the disease. Just to give an example, no longer do we think leprosy is an evil sent to us from afar, for which the only treatment is isolation. We now know it is caused by a bacteria that can be easily killed using the correct antibiotics. We also know that heart attacks are caused by arteries that are clogged by cholesterol and other fats. We know that to prevent heart attacks you have to lower your blood pressure and cholesterol. Obtaining all of this knowledge is nothing short of miraculous. It was such discoveries that made me become a doctor. The scientific process is awe-inspiring: once you identify a disease, you then strive to explain what causes it, and from that you work on a treatment. Such is the case with diabetes. We know why it occurs and how to treat it. However, I have recently noticed a very disturbing trend.

I have noticed that we have all, to some degree or another, started to mistrust medications. Maybe this is a product of the fact that we now all have access to the Internet. Maybe it's all the direct-to-consumer advertising about medications, so most of us are much more knowledgeable about medications than about the diseases they treat. Regardless, I think it is a detrimental trend. I find that way too often my patients ask about the potential side effects of a medication before they ask about the long-term complications of the disease. Unfortunately, I find this to be very common in treating diabetes; one of the first things I hear is: "I don't have to start on insulin, do I?"

I wrote this chapter to demystify the use of medications in treating diabetes. I want you to understand how these medications work so that you can see the reason we sometimes prescribe them. Undoubtedly, trying to treat diabetes with diet and exercise is our main objective. Sometimes, however, there is no choice but to use medications. I don't want you to be afraid of them. I certainly am not. Heck, when I was a kid, it was medications that saved my life.

I was nine years old and living in Detroit, Michigan. Half burned down by the race riots of the previous autumn, Detroit was a cold, dreary, and depressing place. One winter night, I developed severe belly pain. It was excruciating and was accompanied by high fevers and night sweats. Hoping it would go away by itself, I waited two days before I told my parents. By that time it was too late. My appendix had ruptured.

The feces that had been in my appendix had spread throughout my entire abdominal cavity. The infection was life-threatening. Within hours of being examined by a doctor, I was on the operating table. My surgeon did an excellent job of removing my festered appendix and washing out my abdominal cavity, but that was not enough. The infection already established would not go away on its own. To get rid of it, I required intravenous antibiotics for an entire month. After three more months, I was back to my usual self.

I tell you this story because even though a ruptured appendix and type 2 diabetes are vastly different, in many ways the pattern of management for diabetes is a bit like my ruptured appendix and its treatment. The preferred treatment for an infected appendix is to perform a physical act and remove it surgically. The preferred treatment for type 2 diabetes is also to *do something*—in the case of diabetes, it is to change our way of eating and to increase our exercise. In both cases you can take care of the disease by *doing something.* That is, of course, unless the situation has gotten too far along. In the case of my appendix, I had to take antibiotics along with the surgery. Sometimes, in the case of diabetes, you have to take medications along with diet and exercise.

If you have type 2 diabetes, as well intentioned as you may be in trying to achieve control of your blood sugar without using medication, sometimes it just may not be possible. For example, your pancreas may be so depleted of insulin that no amount of exercise can compensate for that deficit. You may need to be on medication that causes your pancreas to release whatever insulin may remain. Please don't think of medication as the enemy. Any medication used to treat diabetes has been researched exhaustively and has been proven to help decrease elevated blood glucose significantly more than a placebo. The potential side effects have also been documented and found to be minor and well below a certain percentage. Medication is not the enemy; on the contrary, it is often a vital part of the cure. It is diabetes that is the enemy. Don't forget that.

We are very lucky to live in an age where we understand the causes of most diseases. Once we understand the mechanics of a disease, it is much easier to figure out how to treat it. With research and advanced statistical techniques, we can further see whether these treatments actually do save and improve lives more than just a sugar pill or placebo. It has been conclusively proven that the early and aggressive treatment of diabetes not only prolongs life but also improves the quality of life. So if you have diabetes, the time to start conquering the illness is *today.* If the healing requires medication, then so be it.

Taking medications to control your diabetes will not only prolong your life, but it will also let you live a healthier life, with a decreased risk of heart attacks, blindness, kidney failure, impotence, and countless other complications of diabetes. Medication can also save your life. This chapter will help you understand more about the medications that treat diabetes and why they are important to you. Knowledge is power. Knowledge also decreases or completely erases fear. If you've never had to take a long-term medication, right now the idea of taking diabetes medications probably seems scary and full of many imaginary dangers. In the pages that follow, we shine a light on these medications so that you realize not only that there is nothing to fear about them, but also that indeed they may well be lifesavers.

DIABETES MEDICATIONS

Diabetes medications are as different as the people who take them. Some people are diagnosed with prediabetes and have no other complications. Some people are diagnosed as full-blown diabetics and have heart attack risk factors such as high cholesterol or high blood pressure. Some people are slightly overweight. Some are already having symptoms from their diabetes, including kidney failure and visual problems. These are just a few of the scenarios that may present when someone is initially diagnosed with type 2 diabetes. There are countless others.

The treatment of diabetes with medication is very individualized and depends on a person's age, how long she has had the disease, whether she has any diabetes complications, how high her blood glucose and A1C are, and many other factors. It is not my intention to provide you with a cookie-cutter treatment formula with this book. Deciding which drug to use first and when is between you and your physician.

For example, I may start a thirty-year-old man with an A1C of 6.5 on a regimen of diet and exercise. However, since there is evidence that starting treatment early may decrease future complications, another physician may immediately start the patient on medication. There are general guidelines recommended by different societies of diabetic specialists, but these guidelines vary a little bit. Suffice to say, however, that if diet and exercise do not work or are not appropriate, a physician will likely start you on an oral medication.

The gold standard of this medication is called metformin (see page 80). If after three months or so, the A1C has not decreased significantly, the physician will either increase the dose of metformin or add a second medication. Usually doctors like to maximize the dose of one medication before adding a second one. In most cases, the second medication is another pill, but in some cases, the second medication is an injectable (non-insulin) medication (injectibles can be easier for the body to absorb). It's not unusual to be on a pill *and* a non-insulin injection. However, if all else fails, a physician may recommend that all oral medication be stopped and you be started on insulin.

What I want you to understand is that diabetes medications work differently. Some draw out insulin from your pancreas. Others cause the insulin you *do* produce to be much more efficient. Sometimes it makes sense to combine one medication from both of these groups. Still other types of medication cause your body to make less glucose or absorb fewer carbohydrates. I don't expect you to understand in a few pages what it took me years of medical school and practice to understand. But if you have a working knowledge of these medications, you can be a more active participant in your care.

This chapter divides diabetes medications into three general categories: oral medications, injectable non-insulin medications, and insulin, including mixed insulins. We doctors *love* to categorize because it makes unfamiliar things easier to understand. We explain how the most common diabetes medications work, and we don't shy away from listing potential side effects. Please note that these possibly harmful symptoms are very infrequent, but you should still be aware of them so you can call your doctor if you experience one.

Knowing about these medications does not mean that *you* should decide which one is best for you. It is your doctor's job to do that. As a matter of fact, a lot of research has gone into analyzing which is the best medication to use, depending on the state of the patient's diabetes. All of these recommendations have been scientifically proven. It *is* your job, however, to know about the medications so that you can ask your health professional any questions or voice any concerns you may have about them. Success in treating diabetes is best achieved using a team approach; I'm just giving you your shoulder pads, helmet, and playbook.

Oral Medications

You already know that type 2 diabetes is basically your body not making sufficient insulin or not responding effectively to the insulin that it *does* produce. Oral diabetes medications work in one or more of the following ways:

- They help your pancreas release more insulin.
- They make your body respond more efficiently to the insulin that your pancreas *does* produce.
- They decrease the amount of glucose produced by your liver.
- They decrease the amount of sugar absorbed in your gut.
- They cause your kidneys to secrete excess glucose.

Whichever way your particular prescription works, the end result is the same: the amount of glucose floating in your blood is lowered. The following are the most common types of oral diabetes medications.

BIGUANIDES

Generic Example: metformin

Brand Names: Glucophage, Glucophage XR, Glumetza, Riomet, Fortamet

HOW IT WORKS:

- Inhibits an enzyme in the liver that decreases the production of glucose in the liver by one-third. The exact molecular mechanism is beyond the scope of this book, but because people with type 2 diabetes produce three times more glucose in the liver than nondiabetics, the use of these drugs makes a big difference in lowering blood sugar levels.

- Antagonizes the action of a hormone called glucagon, which raises blood sugar, especially in between meals. By restricting the action of glucagon, it further decreases fasting blood sugar levels.

- Increases the body's sensitivity to insulin. This make the insulin that *is* produced, even if there is less of it, much more efficient.

- Enhances the use of glucose by peripheral tissues (muscles, brain, heart, and so on), which ultimately removes sugar from the blood.

- Decreases the amount of glucose that is absorbed from the gastro-intestinal tract, thereby not allowing all the carbs that you eat to be absorbed.

BENEFITS:

- Has multiple ways of functioning and is therefore very effective for many different types of people with type 2 diabetes, whether they are overweight, obese, thin, or in between.

- Less likely to cause weight gain than other anti-diabetes medications.

- Less likely to cause excessively low blood sugar (hypoglycemia).

MOST COMMON POTENTIAL SIDE EFFECTS:

- Nausea.

- Diarrhea/bloating.

- Rarely, lactic acidosis.

- Cannot be used by people who have kidney problems. Remind your health care provider that you are on this drug if you have any radiology tests that use dyes, because these can worsen kidney function.

SUMMARY: This is currently the "big daddy" of all anti-diabetes medications. Metformin, a specific type of Biguanides, has quickly become the "go-to" medication to treat diabetes. It is often the first medication used in the treatment of type 2 diabetes, especially in overweight people. It has been shown to have a low probability of causing weight gain and hypoglycemia (low blood sugar). In fact, some studies have suggested that this drug may be protective against cancer.

One of metformin's minor inconveniences is that it must be taken two or three times a day. It can be used alone or in conjunction with other diabetes medications.

In most cases, your doctor will start you off with a metformin-like drug. Only if that doesn't do the work to lower your blood sugar will another class of drug be added. Likewise, if the two don't work, a combination of three might be tried. If the combination is not effective, your physician will probably prescribe insulin.

NOTE: There is a fairly new school of medical thought that believes insulin should be one of the first drugs prescribed rather than the last. Arguments for are that it immediately takes care of elevated blood sugar. Some physicians worry, however, that it may reduce the efficacy of the pancreas that is still producing insulin, and that it may be harder to take the patient off insulin if he loses weight and improves other lifestyle factors. Again, deciding which medications to use and when has to be individualized to the patient and is part of the art of being a physician.

SULFONYLUREAS

Generic Examples: glipizide, glyburide, glimepiride, chlorpropamide, tolazamide, acetohexamide

Brand Names: Glucotrol, Diabinese, Amaryl, Glynase, Diabeta, Glipizide XL, Tolinase, Dymelor, Glucotrol XL, Glycron, Glynase PresTab, Orinase, Tol-Tab

HOW IT WORKS: Sulfonylureas are one of the anti-diabetes classes that have been around for the longest time. Unlike many of the other diabetes medications, which function by helping you metabolize the sugar in your blood, this class actually stimulates the pancreas to manufacture more insulin.

BENEFITS:
- Works rather quickly, often lowering your A1C within a matter of weeks.
- Effective; can lower your A1C by roughly one point.

MOST COMMON POTENTIAL SIDE EFFECTS:
- Low blood sugar. Unlike insulin, which lasts for only a matter of hours in your bloodstream, this class of medication can last for days in your system. If you get hypoglycemia (low blood sugar) while on insulin, you merely have to eat a food that is very high in carbohydrates (juice, for example) and stop taking the insulin. Your blood sugar will quickly return to normal; within minutes you will feel better, and within hours you will be out of danger. With sulfonylureas, however, you run the danger of having repeated episodes of hypoglycemia for days until the medication is out of your system.
- Weight gain.
- Nausea.
- Skin rash.

SUMMARY: This is a tried-and-true medication with many years of clinical experience behind it. But remember: you must not go for extended periods of time without eating while on a sulfonylurea.

MEGLITINIDES

Generic Examples: repaglinide, nateglinide
Brand Names: Prandin, Starlix

HOW IT WORKS: Much like the sulfonylureas, this group works by increasing the amount of insulin manufactured by the pancreas.

BENEFITS: The meglitinides work very quickly; a noticeable drop in A1C can be seen in a matter of weeks.

MOST COMMON POTENTIAL SIDE EFFECTS:
- Severe hypoglycemia
- Weight gain
- Back pain
- Headache

SUMMARY: This is a good class of drug to be used in conjunction with another blood sugar–lowering agent. The same precautions that were expressed with the sulfonylureas concerning hypoglycemia apply here.

DIPEPTIDYL PEPTIDASE-4 (DDP-4) INHIBITORS

Generic Examples: saxagliptin, sitagliptin, linagliptin, alogliptin

Brand Names: Januvia, Onglyza, Tradjenta, Nesina

HOW IT WORKS: This class of medications works in a dual fashion, increasing the amount of insulin produced in the pancreas and decreasing the amount of glucose made in the liver. Therefore, there is more insulin secreted into the bloodstream and less glucose from the liver: a double whammy to lower the overall blood glucose.

BENEFITS: This category of diabetes medication usually does not cause weight gain.

MOST COMMON POTENTIAL SIDE EFFECTS:
- Increased association with upper respiratory infections
- Sore throat
- Headache
- Inflammation of the pancreas (pancreatitis)

SUMMARY: This class of medication is efficient and potent, but beware if you start having severe pain in the upper part of the abdomen that does not go away for hours. Call your physician and report these symptoms; it might be pancreatitis, and *that* can be very dangerous.

THIAZOLIDINEDIONES

Generic Examples: rosiglitazone, pioglitazone, troglitazone

Brand Names: Avandia, Actos, Rezulin

HOW IT WORKS:
- Improves the sensitivity of muscles and fat cells to the insulin that is being produced by the pancreas; that is, increases sensitivity to insulin.

- Decreases the amount of glucose released by the liver.
- Basically, it causes less glucose to be poured into your bloodstream from the liver and allows the insulin that you make to be more efficient in using the glucose in your blood.

BENEFITS: Slightly increases the HDL (good) cholesterol in your body, which in turn decreases your risk of heart disease.

MOST COMMON POTENTIAL SIDE EFFECTS:
- Increased risk of heart attack
- Increased risk of cerebral vascular disease (stroke)
- Associated with liver disease

SUMMARY: The story on this family of medications is a bit mixed. They have been shown to improve your cholesterol levels, but they should be used with caution if you have a history of heart disease, liver disease, or stroke. If you are on one of these and are concerned, do not stop the medication without first consulting your healthcare professional.

ALPHA-GLUCOSIDASE INHIBITORS

Generic Examples: acarbose, miglitol

Brand Names: Glyset, Precose

HOW IT WORKS: This class of drugs works by slowing the digestion, and thus the absorption, of some starches and sugars from your small intestines into the bloodstream. They should be taken with the first bite of a meal. If you are not eating, they should not be taken.

BENEFITS: They don't usually cause weight gain.

MOST COMMON POTENTIAL SIDE EFFECTS:
- Increased production of gas, because these compounds interfere with the breakdown of certain sugars
- Abdominal pain caused by excess gas in the intestines
- Diarrhea/soft feces

SUMMARY: These medications may be a good adjunct to other diabetes medications.

SODIUM GLUCOSE CO-TRANSPONDER 2 INHIBITOR

Generic Examples: canagliflozin, dapagliflozin

Brand Names: Invokana, Farxiga

HOW IT WORKS: These newest oral medications to treat type 2 diabetes work in a completely different way from any other oral diabetes medication. They inhibit the reabsorption of glucose from the kidneys back into the blood stream, thereby causing the glucose to stay in the kidneys and be excreted in the urine. You end up with much glucose in the urine.

BENEFITS:
- Only one pill a day.
- May cause weight loss.
- Some studies show that this drug works very well with metformin, but is still considered a third-line drug to treat type 2 diabetes

MOST COMMON POTENTIAL SIDE EFFECTS:
- Dehydration due to excessive urination
- Hypokalemia (low blood potassium levels)
- Increase in vaginal and penile yeast infections
- People with kidney damage or on dialysis should not take this medication

SUMMARY: These were relatively new medications when we sent this book to press. Therefore, clinical experience is relatively limited. However, these medications look very promising, especially when used in conjunction with other medications.

Injectable Non-Insulin Medications

In my experience, nothing scares a diabetic patient more than having to inject him or herself with a medication, especially if that medication is insulin. There's some sort of psychological barrier for many people that goes beyond just the fear of the needle. It's as if having to take insulin or an injectable medication proves that you have diabetes. There is also the belief that injecting yourself with a medication means going past the point of no return—that you are now stuck forever with having to inject yourself. This is incorrect, but I get it. It's the same reaction that many people have with their medications for other conditions, such as the hypertensive patient who refuses to take his blood pressure medicine or the woman with high cholesterol who does not take her statin pills.

Taking insulin or other injectable medications may be just what the doctor ordered to save your life. The injectable medications that follow are available for the treatment of diabetes. Some are insulin, but the majority are not insulin. They increase the secretion or the efficiency of insulin. However, they still must be given in the form of an injection because the compound would be destroyed by the digestive enzymes found in our gut.

AMYLIN MEMETICS

Generic Example: pramlintide

Brand Names: Symlin

HOW IT WORKS: This class of non-insulin injectable medication slows the passage of food through the intestines, creating a more manageable absorption of carbohydrates. It helps keep after-meal glucose levels from going too high. It also stimulates the release of insulin from the pancreas and reduces the production of glucose from the liver. This medication is very often used in conjunction with insulin injections. However, it cannot be mixed in the same syringe as insulin.

BENEFITS:
- Easily controlled; the correct dosage can be calculated simply.
- May suppress hunger.
- May promote a modest amount of weight loss.

MOST COMMON POTENTIAL SIDE EFFECTS:
- Severely low blood sugar
- Nausea (*Note:* Starting with a low dose and increasing to the maximally beneficial dose can greatly reduce nausea. Be sure to consult with your physician. Do not change your dosage without physician approval.)
- Vomiting
- Headache
- Redness and irritation at the injection site

INCRETIN MIMETICS

Generic Examples: examatide, liraglutide

Brand Names: Byetta, Victoza, Bydureon

HOW IT WORKS: These non-insulin injectable drugs work by stimulating the release of insulin from the pancreas. They also decrease the production of glucose in the liver. These medications are also available in an extended-release formula that can be taken once a week. However, this medication is *not* a substitute for insulin. It should *not* be used in patients with type 1 diabetes or anyone suffering from diabetic ketoacidosis.

BENEFITS:
- May suppress hunger
- Possible weight loss

MOST COMMON POTENTIAL SIDE EFFECTS:
- Nausea
- Vomiting
- Dizziness
- Headache
- Kidney damage or failure
- Hypoglycemia (low blood sugar); especially likely if combined with another type of anti-diabetes medication, such as the sulfonylureas

Insulin

Insulin is the key to controlling diabetes. Lack of insulin or resistance to it causes diabetes. Administration of effective insulin provides an ultimate solution. As you already understand, diabetes is caused when the body does not make enough insulin or the insulin that it *does* make cannot do its work in transporting sugar from the bloodstream to the body's cells. There may come a point in your diabetic experience when you have tried diet and exercise, and even oral medications, and nothing improves your blood sugar sufficiently. This doesn't mean you have done something wrong. It is just your genetic makeup and your current physical state. In cases like these, insulin is needed.

The differences in insulin types have to do with three characteristics:

- How quickly the insulin starts to work after injection
- When the insulin reaches peak efficiency after injection
- How long the insulin lasts in your system after injection

Remember, in the perfect human body, insulin is released by the beta cells of the pancreas within minutes of eating. Sometimes, just the sight and smell of food can trigger this release. This insulin then lasts in the body for a few hours. By using different types of injected insulins with varying times of peak potency, we try to mimic the body's natural response.

Which type of insulin is used depends on both the patient and the doctor. Some patients are unable or unwilling to inject themselves more than once or twice a day. In that case, a slow-acting insulin alone that lasts all day may be preferred. This, however, is not the ideal way of taking insulin, because you miss a lot of the glucose peaks that occur after eating. Ideally, insulin should be injected every minute in response to your blood glucose, just like a normal pancreas would secrete it. That is unrealistic (or is it?). Who wants to give themselves that many injections?

One solution is a combination of slow- and fast-acting insulins. To have as natural an insulin response as possible, some patients are placed on a base of a slow insulin, then asked to measure their blood sugar on a regular basis and give themselves additional fast-acting insulin a few times a day. The amount of fast-acting insulin depends on the blood sugar, measured by a finger-stick blood test. It can be a lot of work, but it is a much more natural way of insulin administration.

The ultimate solution appears to be an insulin pump that continuously monitors your blood sugar level and injects the correct amount of insulin in response to the levels it senses. In other words, an external artificial pancreas. Such devices are already in use. They require surgical implantation of both an insulin holding device and a blood sugar measuring device. Until the day arrives when such a machine is very safe and affordable, we must mimic the pancreas as best we can. This means measuring your blood sugar a few times a day and taking an amount of insulin that corresponds to that measurement. That is why it is so important to understand which type of insulin you may be taking and why. Here are the groups of insulin currently available commercially.

RAPID-ACTING INSULIN

Generic Examples: insulin aspart, insulin lispro, insulin glulisine

Brand Names: Novolog, Apidra, Humolog

ONSET OF ACTION: 15 minutes. Best to inject just before you eat, but beware if you're at a restaurant and you think you can inject as soon as you order. You can't know how long it will take; make sure the food is in front of you before you inject.

PEAK ACTIVITY: 30 to 90 minutes after injection

DURATION OF ACTIVITY: 3 to 5 hours

SHORT-ACTING INSULIN

Generic Example: regular (R)

Brand Names: Novolin R, Humulin R

ONSET OF ACTION: 30 to 60 minutes. Inject almost immediately or up to a maximum of 15 minutes before eating.

PEAK ACTIVITY: 2 to 4 hours

DURATION OF ACTIVITY: 5 to 8 hours

INTERMEDIATE-ACTING INSULIN

Generic Example: NPH (N)

Brand Names: Humulin N, Novolin N

ONSET OF ACTION: 1 to 3 hours

PEAK ACTIVITY: 8 hours

DURATION OF ACTIVITY: 12 to 16 hours

INSULIN PUMPS

A continuous subcutaneous insulin infusion, or an insulin pump, is an amazing device and an excellent way of treating type 1 diabetes. With this type of treatment, a diabetic's blood sugar is constantly measured by a machine, which continually releases insulin subcutaneously (under the skin) without the patient having to do anything. In other words, it does exactly what the pancreas should be doing. However, it is a bit cumbersome. You have to wear a machine all the time, and there is a needle device stuck into your body at all times measuring your blood sugar. All that said, an insulin pump can be miraculous in treating type 1 diabetes. However, is an insulin pump the correct treatment for type 2 diabetes?

The reason this is a question at all is that type 1 and type 2 diabetes are two different animals. As you know, type 1 diabetes is caused by a decrease in (or lack of) insulin production by the pancreas. It makes sense that giving your body insulin constantly is the best treatment. It is almost like having a replacement pancreas—almost. However, especially with obese patients, type 2 diabetes manifests mainly because of the body's resistance to the insulin that *is* produced. Later in the life of some type 2 diabetics, there is a decrease in insulin production that serves only to make treatment more difficult. That explains the need for some people with type 2 diabetes to move from strictly oral medications to injectable medications like insulin. Does it make sense to have insulin constantly pumped into your bloodstream if the body is going to be resistant to it? This is a great question and a highly debated one.

The bottom line is this: we are not sure. (Don't you love science sometimes?) There are currently only two countries in the world that allow insurance reimbursement for insulin pumps as a treatment for type 2 diabetes: France and Israel. There are very few studies that have looked at a large enough number of people to reach a conclusion; plus, the current studies do not always reach the same conclusion. However, one small study did show that for patients with type 2 diabetes who have been having difficulty lowering their A1C with insulin injections, using an external insulin pump was significantly better. This study has not been reproduced in large numbers yet. More research is definitely needed in this field.

All that being said, if I had type 2 diabetes and my doctor and I had tried everything—including diet, exercise, oral medications, and injectable insulin—and *nothing* helped lower my A1C, I would definitely want to try an insulin pump.

Generic Examples: detemir, glargine

Brand Names: Lantus, Levemir

ONSET OF ACTION: 1 hour

PEAK ACTIVITY: Does not peak; has a long, even period of effectiveness

DURATION OF ACTIVITY: 20 to 26 hours

Mixed Insulins

There are now a host of insulin products that come premixed with a combination of insulins that act at different rates. The benefits of these are that you need to take fewer injections and they control your sugar more naturally because the insulin is present in your body before you even eat. However, I recommend these only after you have been on a series of different insulins for a very long time (months or a few years) without varying your dosage. The danger with these mixed insulins is that if you have a day in which you eat much less than you do normally or you exercise much more than usual, you may metabolize your carbohydrates much more quickly. Because there is already a precalculated amount of insulin in your body, your blood sugar may drop dramatically. If this is a type of insulin that you might want to consider, be sure to ask you doctor whether it is right for you.

• • •

Medication is very often an essential and lifesaving part of the treatment of type 2 diabetes. Sure, we all want to heal ourselves naturally, but what is more natural than living a long, healthy life? If that means taking medication, then so be it. Do not be afraid of medications. Just like the antibiotics that saved my life when my appendix ruptured, diabetes medications—when used correctly—will help extend and possibly save your life if you have intractably high blood sugar.

CHAPTER 6

UNDERSTANDING GESTATIONAL DIABETES

ET'S START OFF with this fact: every pregnant woman should be screened for gestational diabetes, no matter what her medical history or state of health. If you've been diagnosed with gestational diabetes, this chapter will give you some good advice and guidelines to follow. If you know someone who is pregnant and you want her to be as healthy as possible during pregnancy, the knowledge you gain from this chapter may be the best gift you can share with her. If you're pregnant and don't know whether you have gestational diabetes, I hope what you read will spur you to get your blood sugar tested.

WHAT IS GESTATIONAL DIABETES?

Gestational diabetes (GDM) appears transiently during pregnancy. It shows itself as elevated blood sugar in women who do not normally have an issue with diabetes. And just as with ordinary type 2 diabetes, GDM indicates that the body is not producing enough insulin or is not responding well to the insulin that is available, so sugar builds up in the blood, while the body is deprived of the fuel it needs. Of course, with the increased weight, including fat, that comes with pregnancy, all of these factors are exaggerated. Nourishing a baby requires so much extra nutrition that the mother's body has to produce more than two hundred times its normal insulin to keep up. But if the pancreas cannot manufacture enough, or the body doesn't respond to the insulin that is produced, the sugar goes unused and remains circulating in the blood.

Why hyperglycemia may develop suddenly during pregnancy is not fully understood. Recent studies suggest that it may be triggered by hormones and metabolic changes in the mother. Hormones in the developing placenta, in particular, are designed to block the action of insulin so there is more nourishment circulating in the blood to feed the fetus. With GDM, this insulin resistance gets out of hand.

Gestational diabetes usually disappears after the baby is born. However, even one bout is predictive of a much greater risk of regular type 2 diabetes five to ten years down the line. Fully 35 percent of women with GDM will at some point go on to develop type 2 diabetes. So if you've had this problem during pregnancy, regular screening for elevated blood sugar at least every three years is highly advised.

GDM also predicts a greater chance of a recurrence during a subsequent pregnancy. Perhaps most important, if not discovered and treated appropriately, the condition can have profound negative repercussions for the birth, the baby, and even your child's health later in life. And it's not a rare condition. Fully 15 to 20 percent of pregnant women develop gestational diabetes in varying degrees of severity.

If you're overweight or obese, you are at greater risk. Living a sedentary lifestyle—not exercising or being physically active—being over twenty-five years of age, or having a family history of the disease also increases your odds. GDM is more common in African American, Hispanic, and Native American women—the same ethnic groups that suffer from more type 2 diabetes. Whether this ethnic disparity is due to genetic factors or lifestyle conditions, we don't yet know. But it's important to keep the statistics in mind so that you are aware of your risk and respond to it appropriately. That means if you come from a background at higher risk of developing diabetes, it's all the more important to watch your diet, stay physically active, and make sure you are screened regularly.

For the baby, the risks are serious and long term. The fetus absorbs all this extra sugar circulating in the mother's body through the placenta, but the mother's insulin does not accompany it. Consequently, the developing baby's pancreas is forced to overproduce insulin to try and keep up with the excess sugar it's getting from the mother. So in essence, the baby is overfed in the womb.

The result is an abnormally large newborn, meaning the baby weighs more than 9 pounds at birth compared to an average healthy birth weight of 6½ to 8 pounds. There was a time when we boasted of a baby's hefty weight with pride. But you can have too much of a good thing. An infant who is overweight makes for a traumatic birth—for mother and child. Physical damage to the shoulders during birth and acute breathing problems shortly after birth are two issues that often arise. Because many of these large-at-birth (macrosomial) babies have to be delivered by Cesarean section, complications associated with such a surgery, such as infections and persistent bleeding, can also occur.

Another major risk for the baby is low blood sugar (hypoglycemia) because of the overproduction of insulin, which can be life threatening. Infants with low blood sugar after birth may not have any symptoms. Therefore, the hospital nurse should check the infant's blood sugar level often. If symptoms do occur, there may be irritability, problems keeping warm, blue-colored skin, tremors, shakiness, and seizures, to name but a few.

More profound, perhaps, are recent studies that suggest that the birth weight of the baby can have consequences throughout the child's life. An overweight baby is much more likely to become an obese adult and to develop type 2 diabetes. Again, we don't know why this is the case. It may have

RISK FACTORS FOR GESTATIONAL DIABETES

- Carrying too much weight. Being obese—having a BMI of 30 kg/m² or higher—is associated with even higher risk than being overweight (having a BMI between 25 and 29.9 kg/m²).
- Being of African American, Hispanic, or Native American heritage.
- Getting pregnant after the age of twenty-five; women over thirty-five are at significantly higher risk.
- Having a family history of type 2 diabetes.
- Having a personal history of prediabetes or having suffered from gestational diabetes during a previous pregnancy.
- Previously having given birth to a baby nine pounds or heavier.

something to do with early hormone signaling or problems with the establishment of the proper gut bacteria, but whatever the cause, we have enough statistics to know it is true. So losing weight before you get pregnant, taking care of yourself during your pregnancy, and especially making sure you are tested for gestational diabetes, all can have long-term benefits for your baby.

SCREENING FOR GESTATIONAL DIABETES

Historically, screening for GDM was left up to the individual obstetrician. Different doctors had different ideas about when to test or whether to test at all. Recently, however, the importance of identifying GDM was recognized, given that one in five pregnant women develops gestational diabetes. And just as with type 2 diabetes, many have no overt symptoms. So no matter the woman's weight or family history, the advice now is to screen all pregnant women for gestational diabetes at between twenty-four and twenty-eight weeks of pregnancy. If your health care professional doesn't suggest testing you, you should ask about it. It's good to know the tests and the numbers, so you can understand your own results.

To be screened for gestational diabetes, at roughly twenty-six weeks, you'll be given a 50-gram oral glucose challenge test. This involves drinking 50 grams of pure glucose dissolved in water and seeing what happens to your blood sugar. Of course, right after drinking pure sugar syrup, everyone's blood sugar spikes. But after an hour, it should be less than 140 mg/dl. If it's 140 or higher, the doctor will order a second test to make sure of the diagnosis. The reason for the second test is that any pregnant woman might have some insulin resistance or elevated blood sugar because her body is in a heightened state designed to feed the developing baby.

The second test comprises a simple fasting plasma blood test (see page 23) followed by a 100-gram oral glucose tolerance test (see page 24). You drink an even sweeter beverage, and small amounts of blood are drawn at regular intervals. The results of both tests are calculated, and if any two of the following results are evident, you'll be considered positive for gestational diabetes:

- Before drinking the glucose: fasting plasma glucose > 95 mg/dl
- One hour after the challenge: plasma glucose > 180 mg/dl
- Two hours after the challenge: plasma glucose > 155 mg/dl
- Three hours after the challenge: plasma glucose > 140 mg/dl

Once you've been diagnosed, you'll work with your doctor on treatment. Unlike a diabetic who has months to correct her blood sugar, a woman with gestational diabetes needs to move quickly. Every day is important in fetal development, so normalization of the blood glucose must happen right away.

YOU'VE BEEN DIAGNOSED WITH GESTATIONAL DIABETES

First of all, don't panic. Now is *not* the time to go on a crash diet, but a diagnosis can provide a major wake-up call for improving your diet and exercise habits. Reducing the amount of sugar and starch in your diet will help greatly, but you must also follow a diet that will allow appropriate weight gain and at the same time provide the nutrients you and your baby need to thrive. Your main goal is to maintain blood sugar levels that are normal throughout your pregnancy in order to ensure healthy fetal development. Although this isn't the time to lose weight, you should gain weight in a measured, appropriate manner with an appropriate diet.

The same types of foods recommended for type 2 diabetics are helpful for gestational diabetes—that is, carbohydrates with a low glycemic index (see page 108), moderate protein, enough dairy, and lots of vegetables. Because you are also supporting your growing baby, your portions may be larger for some food groups, such as dairy, so consult with your doctor or a registered dietitian nutritionist for specifics. Proper nutrition will help avoid low blood sugar and getting enough fluids and fiber, in particular, will alleviate some of the unpleasant gastrointestinal symptoms associated with any pregnancy, including heartburn, nausea, and constipation.

Stepping up your physical activity, with medical approval, will also help control your blood sugar. The combination of a healthy diet and moderate exercise may even prevent the need for you to take insulin or allow for smaller dosages. However, if your blood sugar remains uncontrolled, you will need to take insulin. Insulin has been the gold standard of treatment for GDM for many decades now. But it, too, has its issues: bouts of hypoglycemia, constant injections, and the fact that women taking insulin tend to gain even more weight.

Metformin (see page 80) has been found to be a safe alternative for treating GDM. One of the main reasons is that metformin improves insulin sensitivity and has less associated weight gain. This is quite advantageous during pregnancy. There is also evidence that metformin can reduce the risk of preeclampsia (dangerously high blood pressure during pregnancy) and the need for Cesarean sections because the baby is too large. As always, please consult your physician. It is essential that you follow the regimen your doctor prescribes and take your medication exactly as recommended. Chances are you'll be able to go off any prescribed medication as soon as your baby is born.

We have come a long way in being able to identify and treat gestational diabetes. And although the main treatment is diet and exercise, the best solution is to avoid developing it in the first place.

PREVENTING GESTATIONAL DIABETES

Of all the risk factors for gestational diabetes, the only one over which you truly have control is your weight. The best way to prevent gestational diabetes is to get your weight under control *before* you get pregnant. When you are nurturing a developing baby inside your body, it's not the time to diet. That prepregnancy weight loss must go hand in hand with sound nutrition, because fad diets that restrict major food groups are not sound for your health or your future baby's health.

The Blood Sugar Budget (see chapter 8) is an excellent program designed to provide you with a low-glycemic-index diet containing all the nutrients you need while promoting healthy weight loss. In this plan we recommend you eat as many vegetables as you can—raw and lightly cooked—and opt for chicken or fish over red meat, including pork. Green vegetables like kale, broccoli, collards, brussels sprouts, and Swiss chard provide many minerals and vitamins, including folate, which is essential for preventing certain birth defects. You also need to get enough calcium. Dairy products—including cheese and yogurt—are rich sources of calcium, as are soy milk, salmon, and bone-in sardines. And moderate amounts of extra-virgin olive oil should be your fat of choice.

As delicious as our recipes are (see chapter 9), you will probably have to give up some foods that may be old favorites: fried foods, sweets, cakes, cookies, chips, and sugary sodas, including diet sodas. Many colas contain a chemical that some studies have associated with cancer, and when you are pregnant or preparing to be, you want to eat as pure a diet as possible. And sodas filled with artificial sweeteners go hand in hand with weight gain.

Before getting pregnant, switch to a healthier way of eating, like that suggested by our Blood Sugar Budget, to lose weight slowly and steadily. We make sure you get all the nutrients you need to maintain good health, lower your blood sugar, and improve your insulin resistance. We also set you up to get the right nutrition for you and your baby when you do become pregnant.

Once you get pregnant, you don't want to continue to lose weight, but you should gain weight only at a controlled rate. Your doctor or nurse will either counsel you or refer you to a qualified registered dietitian nutritionist to tell you how much weight you should gain and when. Unfortunately, being pregnant is not a license to eat everything in sight. Understand just how much weight you should gain each trimester, and try not to gain a single pound more than is prescribed. Most pregnant women on average need only 300 extra calories a day; that's not a lot. And studies have shown that babies born to women who gain more than forty pounds during pregnancy have a much greater likelihood of ending up obese, even in their teens. Gaining only the appropriate weight and eating a healthy low-glycemic diet for even just a month reduces your chances of developing gestational diabetes.

There is also substantial evidence that exercise can help prevent or actually cure gestational diabetes. We know that along with healthy weight, maintaining regular moderate physical activity is key to all good health but especially important for insulin sensitivity, which affects blood sugar levels.

It's best to start your exercise program before you get pregnant. Introducing anything new and strenuous early in pregnancy is not a good idea. But you can start slowly and build up. There are exercise programs designed expressly for pregnant women, which make sure all the positions and postures are safe. And you can always begin a regular walking practice, which benefits almost everyone. Comfortable shoes with rubber soles and good ankle support are a good investment to prevent slipping or tripping. Check with your doctor to make sure your physical activity choices are healthy for you and your baby.

More and more studies are offering evidence that the health of the mother and what she eats while she is pregnant can have long-lasting influence on her child, not only in the womb and as a newborn, but also throughout the child's lifetime. In fact, some effects caused by the nutrients and/or toxins a pregnant woman is exposed to can carry over to future generations. Now that screening for all pregnant women is the medical standard, gestational diabetes and the risks associated with it don't have to affect your child. Prevention and treatment alike can ensure a healthier mother and a healthier baby.

PART TWO

MANAGE YOUR DIABETES

CHAPTER 7

GOOD FOODS, BAD FOODS: WHAT YOU SHOULD EAT

INVARIABLY, WHEN PEOPLE are diagnosed with prediabetes or type 2 diabetes, the first question they ask is: "What should I eat?" If you scan the Internet or pick up half a dozen books on diabetes, you'll probably see half a dozen different answers: a low-carb, low-fat diet; a low-carb, high-fat diet; a high-protein diet; a low-calorie diet; and so on. How do you know which, if any, are based on sound scientific evidence and, more important, how do you know which one is best for you?

Well, first of all: one reason for the number of choices is that diabetes counseling is not a one-size-fits-all plan. People come in all shapes, sizes, and genetic types; they have their own coexisting diseases; and they respond in unique ways to various foods. That's why, ultimately, you should take this book to your health care professional and use it as a base for your own personalized diabetes diet. But what you will find here, the Blood Sugar Budget, is a great place to start. This simple program incorporates all the latest knowledge about what type of eating plan reduces blood sugar and helps you lose weight and identifies which foods in general are associated with better insulin response and less type 2 diabetes.

THE TRUTH ABOUT FAT

Contrary to popular belief, there are very few completely *good* or *bad* foods. Most of the things we eat are made up of nutrients that are helpful in some ways and not in others. In the past twenty years, we've learned that refined carbohydrates are likely to be worse for us than saturated fats. So now we know not all fat is bad. Very likely in the next few years we'll learn that not all saturated fats are bad, because they come in many forms and compositions. Some of the fat recommendations we make here may surprise you, because the public has been given so much well-intentioned but perhaps misguided nutritional information over the past twenty years. Don't forget, before the dangers of trans fats were discovered, every doctor and nutritionist was pushing margarine over butter.

One saturated fat that seems to be beneficial to people with type 2 diabetes or insulin resistance is dairy fat, because it is rich in a couple of fatty acids, which happen to be saturated, that are associated with better insulin response and less diabetes. A number of large studies have shown benefits from eating dairy foods, and—surprise!—some have shown no benefit from eating low-fat dairy. In fact, some studies have suggested that moderate amounts of full-fat dairy are associated with fewer cases of type 2 diabetes and less risk of cardiovascular disease.

Keep in mind that you can absorb only so much calcium and fat at a time. So I recommend that you have a good source of calcium three times a day, with at least two of those sources coming from small portions of natural, whole-fat dairy: 6 ounces (about ⅔ cup) yogurt or 1 to 1½ ounces (2 to 3 tablespoons) farmstead cheese, preferably one containing live cultures. A teaspoon of heavy cream in coffee in the morning avoids the carbs and sugar in milk and delivers healthy fats at a cost of only 17 calories, if you measure carefully. But of course, large amounts of saturated fats are probably not beneficial, and they contain a lot of calories. That's why portion control is so important.

Note: I don't recommend cow's milk as a beverage, even though it is a rich source of calcium, because it is so high in carbohydrates and sugar. The American Diabetes Association recommends a glass of skim or

Be suspicious of so-called *superfoods*—that is, any one food purported to cure all ills. You'll see them hyped on the Internet and in magazines. But don't you think if there were one food you could eat or one supplement you could swallow that could magically melt off pounds and lower elevated blood sugar to normal levels and keep your brain sharpened like a pencil for life that it would not be a secret? Any number of pharmaceutical companies or manufacturers would have bottled the active ingredient and sold it for a pretty penny. Sure, blueberries are good for you. But eating nothing but blueberries is not practical and would not supply you with all the nutrition you need. Coconut oil, which is all the rage now, is good in some ways. But because it is shorter in length than most fats, it is metabolized in a simpler fashion, which results in faster absorption into the bloodstream. Consequently, eating it regularly can pack on the pounds very quickly.

Don't forget, any time a scientist does a study indicating a food might be good for certain conditions, the marketing teams that sell that food jump on the bandwagon and push it as far as it will go. Think of the lists of foods that have been popular over the years: pomegranate, coconut oil, blueberries, chia seeds, açaì juice. It's not that these foods don't have valuable nutrients to offer, but there's no one food that can solve all your problems. Variety is not only the spice of life, it's also the staff of life.

1 percent milk as an emergency fix if you start feeling faint from hypoglycemia. It's right up there with orange juice and glucose to ramp up your blood sugar quickly. It is also a highly allergic food.

We also need variety in our diet in order to obtain all the necessary nutrients from our food. That's why nutritionists urge people to eat a rainbow plate of food. Each different color in fruits and vegetables or the yellow in the yolk of an egg represent different chemicals that are showing more and more benefits for human health.

Foods are also hugely affected by other foods. If you eat an egg, for example, you're ingesting some very good-quality protein, about 150 mg of cholesterol, and lots of good nutrients in that yolk: B12, biotin, iron, choline, and vitamins A and D. Many of these nutrients are vitamins that are hard to get elsewhere. But if you have a small bowl of oatmeal along with that egg, you'll still obtain all of that good nutrition, but some of that cholesterol will be bound with the soluble fiber in the oatmeal and carried off before your body can absorb it. That's one reason a high-fiber diet can be beneficial for many people.

You may be surprised to learn that we propose the same eating plan for people with prediabetes as for those who have already progressed to type 2 diabetes. This recommendation dovetails with the current evidence: a recent study recommended essentially identical foods for healthy adults as for people diagnosed with diabetes. Healthy eating is healthy eating, though there are conflicting schools of thought about which foods are nutritious. That's because many of our nutritional beliefs are in a state of flux, and recent studies are pointing us in a very different direction from the "low fat" mantra that has proved so ineffectual over the past few decades.

About twenty years ago, the government was facing a population in which 35 percent of people were obese and another 25 percent were overweight—both conditions that put people at much greater risk for developing not only diabetes, but also heart disease, high blood pressure, osteoarthritis, and even cancer. Therefore, the government needed a simple message to promote healthier eating, and they believed the American people could not deal with complexity.

The main message, broadcast far and wide, was that all fat is bad for you—period. Initially, there was no reference to different types of fat. Later on, it was qualified a bit: all fat is bad for you, and saturated fat is terrible. It turns out, the government was wrong on both counts. Its message was inaccurate—some fats, such as monounsaturated fats, are good for you, even necessary—and the American public is smart enough to understand that there may be some good fats and some bad fats. What resulted from this compounding of errors was the fattening of America— with overweight and obesity rates today soaring above 70 percent, and roughly seventy-nine million of these people not even knowing their blood sugar is high.

The misguided scientific information that fat is bad, period, began with the Framingham Heart Study, begun in 1948, a huge, ongoing survey of more than five thousand adult men and women in the town of Framingham, Massachusetts. By following this population over a long period of time, the study attempted to identify which dietary and lifestyle factors contributed the most to cardiovascular disease—heart attack and stroke. These people were evaluated every two years, and in 1971 a second generation was enrolled from adult children of the original cohort and their spouses. This study identified several major risk factors for cardiovascular disease: smoking, obesity, diabetes, physical inactivity, high blood pressure, and high cholesterol. These results were amplified in 1958 by the work of a scientist named Ancel Keys, who surveyed seven countries and concluded that fat and heart disease are inextricably linked. Recently, many people have attacked his findings.

We do know that saturated fat raises cholesterol. That's what led to the huge low-fat campaign of the past few decades, with dietary guidelines that resulted in huge increases in overweight, obesity, and diabetes. An issue that has been raised recently is whether cholesterol caused by higher dietary fat intake actually results in more deaths from heart attack and stroke or not. On this matter, the jury is still out.

Several recent studies have offered compelling evidence that, yes, too much red meat is definitely bad for you, but it has to do with factors other than the saturated fat. On top of that, there are different blends of fatty acids in all fats and oils, and many of the fats in dairy fat may be beneficial, especially for keeping the brain young and staving off Alzheimer's disease and other forms of dementia. It bears repeating: 60 percent of the brain is made up of fat, glucose is its favorite food, and it needs feeding all the time.

THE BLOOD SUGAR BUDGET PREVIEW

So if saturated fat is bad for you, carbs and sweets encourage diabetes, and too much protein may be a strain on your body, what are you supposed to eat? That's what we're here to answer. First of all, not all fats are alike, and not all saturated fats are alike. Most fats are made up of several different kinds of fat. For example, olive oil, which has been shown in numerous studies to be one of the healthiest fats you can eat, is touted for the benefits of its monounsaturated fats. These tend to raise HDL, the good cholesterol. Olive oil also provides many anti-inflammatory antioxidants and polyphenols, which act almost like natural aspirin. But olive oil is also made up of one-third saturated fat.

From previous studies, we already know that people who eat a Mediterranean diet have fewer chronic diseases, including diabetes. A recent controlled trial in Spain showed that people fed the Mediterranean diet, with additional generous amounts of extra-virgin olive oil beyond ordinary use, had 35 percent less risk of cardiovascular disease than people

GLYCEMIC INDEX VERSUS GLYCEMIC LOAD

Glycemic index and *glycemic load* are two terms you'll frequently hear mentioned in connection with blood sugar. Glycemic index is essentially a measure of the power of carbohydrates in a particular food to boost blood sugar. Individual foods are measured against glucose, which has a glycemic index of 100, and white bread, which has a glycemic index of 70. In general, an index number higher than 70 is considered a high-glycemic food; foods that fall in the 55 to 70 range are classified as moderate, and an index of number lower than 55 is relatively low. It seems simple doesn't it?

Unfortunately, nutrition is more complex. Just because a food contains a certain type of carbohydrate doesn't mean your body has access to it. And the portion of the food you would normally consume might be different from that used to measure the index. Also, you rarely eat a single ingredient by itself.

That gets us to glycemic load, another measurement of the power of carbs in food to boost blood sugar. In addition to factoring in the carbohydrates in food, glycemic load also takes into account the amount of food you would normally eat as well as other components that might alter how available the carbohydrates are to affect blood sugar. Everything you eat over the course of a meal, including what you drink, will affect the glycemic load. Therefore, when you have a sweet or starchy snack, it's best to pair it with a modest amount of fat or some protein—both of which will moderate the rise in blood sugar caused by the carbohydrate.

Fiber also causes a big difference between the glycemic index and the glycemic load. Studies have proven that a high-fiber diet helps slow the rise in blood sugar after eating. A carrot, for example, contains a fair amount of sugar, but it's also high in fiber. So while under chemical analysis, a raw carrot has a glycemic index higher than 40, its glycemic load is about 3. That's why we recommend that you eat cereal with at least 5 grams of fiber, or meals loaded with beans, vegetables, and whole grains. Having a lot of fiber in your diet lowers the effect of a higher glycemic food.

Because it considers more factors, glycemic load is a more helpful number to focus on. There is much evidence that a low–glycemic load diet:

- improves blood sugar values
- improves insulin resistance and the ability of the pancreas to secrete insulin
- reduces cholesterol levels and biochemical markers of inflammation
- reduces risk of metabolic syndrome

on a control diet. Since heart disease is a major risk factor for people with diabetes, this has huge significance. Other studies have highlighted the benefits of whole grains, especially cereal grains, and beta glucans, the particular soluble fiber in oatmeal and barley, for decreasing the risk of type 2 diabetes and improving cholesterol profiles for cardiovascular health. And several meta-analyses have shown a 16 percent reduction in type 2 diabetes among people who ate the most leafy green vegetables. Eating a diet low in glycemic index foods (see box opposite) automatically reduces calories. But just counting carbs, like counting calories, can be of dubious benefit, because although some very healthful foods, like beans, are high in carbs, their high-fiber, low-fat profile makes them excellent choices.

Whether you have been diagnosed with prediabetes or type 2 diabetes, the goals are the same: to achieve or maintain a healthy weight, eat nutrient-rich foods (plenty of vegetables, fruit, and whole grains, and avoid added refined sugar, red meat, and processed foods), and tip that bottle of olive oil with a liberal hand. No matter where you look, the Mediterranean diet is consistently associated with less chronic disease—including diabetes and heart disease—and with better weight control and blood pressure.

Of course there are certain foods that should be eaten as seldom as possible, if at all: sweets, refined starches like white bread and white rice, processed meats like bacon and sausage, and saturated meat fats. But even with a lot of lists, choosing what to eat and when can be confusing. The Blood Sugar Budget makes it easy, and many of the foods you are permitted to eat may surprise you. Our program contains a number of foods you probably thought you couldn't eat and advises staying away from some types of foods you may have thought were good for you. Full-fat cheeses and yogurt and fruit in appropriate portions, for example, are part of the program. That's because the dairy contains a particular fatty acid that is associated with less type 2 diabetes and improved insulin response, and the fruit is loaded with polyphenols—chemicals that improve the way the body functions—as well as plenty of fiber.

The bottom line is you don't eat *fats* and *carbs* and *protein*; you eat butter and bread and steak. Or olive oil and oatmeal and salmon. You shouldn't need a degree in biochemistry to figure out what's in food. We've already done that for you. And we've recommended groups of foods in appropriate amounts that will steady your blood sugar, reduce it over time, and help you lose weight.

The Blood Sugar Budget food groups include nonstarchy vegetables, like leafy greens, as well as healthy oils; whole grains; fruits; and lean protein, dairy, beans, and eggs. It's called a "budget" because there is a maximum number of points you are allowed each day, and each of these categories contains different numbers of points. Some foods are free, so you can eat them liberally without worrying about the consequences; others, such as sweet desserts, are pricey and can be afforded only a couple of times a week.

This approach works much better than counting calories and fat. I've seen countless obese diabetic patients who come to see me with their blood sugar out of control and complaining that they cannot lose weight while eating 1,200 calories a day. Almost invariably, they're eating a bagel with cream cheese for breakfast, a muffin for a snack, a sandwich for lunch, and scraps for dinner. And they are drinking a ton of diet sodas. In that kind of diet, there are too many refined carbs, not enough protein, and nothing to nourish the good gut bacteria that regulate carbohydrate and fat metabolism: fiber and healthy oils.

Conquering diabetes means not only understanding what you cannot eat, but also eating foods you *should* eat. It entails spreading out your carbohydrate consumption evenly throughout the day, trying to eat at the same time every day, and not skipping meals. The goal is to set up a metabolic memory, sort of like muscle memory, to help you keep your blood sugar steady and avoid highs and lows.

Well, you may say, *if I really want to avoid insulin spikes and lower my blood sugar, why don't I just stop eating all carbohydrates?* Because if you have type 2 diabetes, your pancreas is still working and your body is set up to accommodate a certain amount of carbohydrates. This is where you get your energy to run the exquisite machine that is your body. A number of studies have shown that the people who do best in terms of controlling blood sugar and avoiding complications are those who eat moderate amounts of carbohydrates, especially whole grains, as well as appropriate fat and fiber so their body can cope with them easily. Don't forget, those same food that contain carbohydrates deliver valuable B vitamins, antioxidants, and, in some cases, protein as well as energy.

We do offer a list of foods that simply are not healthy for you whether you are diabetic or not and should be left off your plate as much as possible. These are foods that are associated with chronic diseases and higher death rates and are worth giving up—even though you may crave them. Ice cream won't kill you, though it can raise your blood sugar and make you fat. Bacon and bologna are filled with nitrates, chemicals that are converted into carcinogenic compounds in the body; they are also linked to greater risk of diabetes. If you can't give them up, at least consider eating them as seldom as possible—for a special occasion once every couple of weeks rather than as a daily staple.

THE RECIPES

In the Blood Sugar Budget, we offer a menu of choices. Broadening your culinary horizons and eating a variety of fruits and vegetables play a large part. To make it easier and more palatable, we also offer more than one hundred recipes to help you choose what to eat for those three meals and two snacks you should have every day.

Many people skip breakfast. However, some studies have shown that larger breakfasts are associated with less weight gain. Keep in mind, an Egg McMuffin has 300 calories. They say that's not much, but at home you could have an egg for 80 calories, a piece of whole grain toast or half of a high-fiber English muffin with a slice of real cheese with fats that have been shown to improve insulin for about 110 calories, and a large wedge of cantaloupe for 60 calories, for a total of 250 calories. That's 50 calories less than that fast-food breakfast sandwich and a whole lot more nutrition, fiber, vitamins, and minerals, and no nitrates.

On the Blood Sugar Budget we offer a number of appetizing breakfast options, as well as an assortment of smoothies, which incorporate vegetables and fruits with a dairy protein source that's handy to take along if you're on the go. Just keep in mind that your body does not respond the same way to liquids as to solids, so the smoothie might be part of a complete breakfast, or a helpful nutritious snack to maintain your blood sugar in the middle of the morning.

We also present an assortment of appetizers and snacks. Most people benefit from spreading out their carbs and calories throughout the day, eating three smaller meals and a couple of modest healthy snacks. It may seem counterintuitive, but eating all this food—rather than taking in 1,200 calories in two or three meals laden with refined carbohydrates and starving yourself the rest of the time—will actually help you lose weight and normalize your blood sugar. I've had many patients say to me, "I can't believe I'm eating all this food and I'm losing weight. And I feel so much better." If you're like most prediabetes and type 2 diabetes patients, your energy is often in short supply and flags late in the morning and in the middle of the afternoon or right after work. That's when these snacks come in: to maintain appropriate blood sugar at a steadier rate so there are fewer spikes of insulin.

Although nuts are healthy, they are extremely high in calories, so while you're losing weight you can have a few in your smoothies or along with half an apple as a snack, but yogurt, fruit, beans, and vegetables are probably better options. Your snack could be as simple as a small apple or half an avocado, or it could consist of one of our wonderful dips with some raw vegetables.

Soups offer a great way to fill up with fluids and extend the pleasure of the meal without adding a lot of calories or fat. We offer a template for a simple soup made with almost any vegetable, ready in twenty minutes or less, as well as some more substantial chunky soups and chowders that, paired with a salad, some whole grain bread, and cheese could make a very nice Sunday supper.

Chicken and turkey as well as fish and shellfish—and tofu if you enjoy it—are the best protein bases of a diabetic diet. Grass-fed free-range beef and lamb, as well as lean cuts of pork are other options, but we recommend they be eaten less frequently—once a week at most. And fatty cuts of meat or processed meats are simply not part of a healthy diet.

A controversy is raging in the medical and scientific community right now about the role saturated fats play in the promotion of disease. There is a dangerous ingredient in red meat (which includes pork, by the way, despite the excellent marketing campaign for "The Other White Meat") but it's not clear it's the saturated fat. A chemical called *carnitine,* which is vital for fatty acid synthesis and essential for health, interacts with the bacteria in your gut, sometimes fermenting into a highly atherosclerotic substance called *trimethylamine N-oxide,* usually referred to as TMAO. A large controlled trial out of the Cleveland Clinic, one of the largest and most respected heart hospitals in the country, showed that regular meat eaters, when fed an 8-ounce steak, registered a huge uptick in TMAO in their blood not long after eating the beef. But when vegetarians or vegans were fed the same steak, no increase was seen. The hypothesis is that different diets produce different gut bacteria, and it is this symbiotic microbiome that mediates what we eat. It's an exciting area of research. It may be a few years before we know for sure whether red meat and/or saturated fat is good, bad, or neutral. In the meantime, striving to eat a more plant-based diet is probably the best choice.

Meats and other major protein sources—fish, poultry, tofu, eggs—do not affect blood sugar significantly, so there is a temptation to opt for a really high-protein diet. But it's important to remember that although we need enough protein, your body can only process so much at a time; the excess is simply peed out or broken down and stored as fat. In the metabolism of protein, a lot of acid is produced, which causes inflammation and can weaken bone composition. When the body is in danger of becoming acidic, a hormone is triggered that breaks down bone to release calcium, which neutralizes acid. So too much protein, especially from powerful sources like red meat, put a strain on the kidneys and potentially weaken bones, leading to osteoporosis.

The Mediterranean diet has been associated with the lowest risk of type 2 diabetes and heart disease, as well as less cancer, obesity, high blood pressure, and even cognitive decline. It entails eating more fruits and vegetables, especially vegetables, as well as whole grains, more fish and chicken than red meat, moderate amounts of wine, and olive oil used liberally as the major fat.

And while most American studies reflexively include "low-fat dairy" as a recommendation, this is a conjecture of the American nutrition establishment to conform to the "low-fat" mantra preached over the past twenty years. In fact, a tour of the Mediterranean countries, from France to Spain, Italy, and as far east as Turkey, or a survey of recipes from these cultures, will show little evidence of "low-fat" diary products. Instead, moderate amounts of full-fat dairy are a major part of the diet in these countries—small wedges of artisanal cheeses and full-fat live culture yogurt, in particular—or a portion of a naturally low-fat cheese like *fromage blanc* in France. A few years ago, a controlled trial out of Denmark showed that cheese did not raise LDL cholesterol, but butter most certainly did.

Whichever dairy is chosen, portions are small. These cultures don't drink milk as a beverage in large quantities. They consume 6 to 8 ounces a day of these natural dairy products. In addition, a number of studies by major researchers in the field have not shown any appreciable benefits of low-fat dairy; in fact, some have shown adverse effects in terms of obesity, which tends to lead to diabetes.

Now that you have some idea of which foods are beneficial for overall good health, weight control, and diabetes management, you need a way to put them all together in a real-life plan. You need to know not only what to eat, but also how much and how often. That's where our Blood Sugar Budget in the next chapter comes in.

CHAPTER 8

THE BLOOD SUGAR BUDGET

IF YOU ARE LIKE ME AND have always fought the battle of the bulge, you must admit that the times you were most able to keep your weight under control were the times you were most conscious about what you were eating. You were aware. You paid attention to what you were consuming instead of bingeing one day and swearing you would make up for it the next. Perhaps you did it on your own by counting calories. Or perhaps you did some sort of program that assigned points to what you ate. Many of those programs work quite well. But new research is being done all the time on diet and health. Findings over the past couple of years have huge ramifications for people who want to eat to lose weight and avoid chronic diseases such as type 2 diabetes at the same time. As a result, we created the Blood Sugar Budget, a nutritional program and way of eating that optimizes your diet for both weight loss and control of blood sugar.

While working toward a healthy weight must be a goal for anyone who has been diagnosed with prediabetes or type 2 diabetes, it's important to keep in mind that following a crash diet to restrict calories is not helpful. As a matter of fact, it is probably counterproductive. Even while you're striving to shave off excess pounds, you still need to keep your blood sugar levels as even as possible. If you avoid all carbohydrates, your body's engine will run out of steam and stimulate sugar production in the liver. But by eating the right carbohydrates spread evenly throughout the day, you help prevent blood sugar levels from spiking. The right carbohydrates are foods like vegetables, beans, fruits, and whole grains, all of which provide fiber and valuable vitamins and minerals along with whatever starches or sugars they contain. And pairing carbs with fat, dairy, or protein can slow the absorption of glucose, fine-tune your metabolism, and optimize your health. We are not suggesting that you starve to control your diabetes; on the contrary, we want to teach you how to eat well and with gusto, but you need to eat the right foods.

While there is no one superfood that will cure everything, there are a number of foods and food groups associated with improved glycemic control, less diabetes, and better health. These foods form the foundation of the Blood Sugar Budget. Every food group listed is there for a reason, and although we recommend serving sizes that are most likely to improve your diabetes or prediabetes, you get to choose what you feel like eating. Remember that old saying that slow and steady wins the race? Well, that's true when it comes to eating a healthy diet as well. Your ultimate goal is to learn a healthier way of eating for the rest of your life. Anyone can lose weight; the hard part is keeping it off. And with a diagnosis of diabetes, it is not just weight management that is important—blood sugar control must be an ongoing priority as well.

UNDERSTANDING THE BUDGET

Here's how it works: The Blood Sugar Budget assigns each type of food a point value. These points correlate to both the nutrients you need to improve your diabetes and the amount of each food that you can eat and still lose weight. If you stick with the prescribed foods and the target number of points, you will most likely lose a pound or two a week, which is what we're aiming for. You are allotted 42 to 50 points per day, or a maximum of 350 points a week. Just as you are obligated to pay your mortgage or rent every month along with your utility, phone, or cable bills, you must spend a certain number of points every day on specially designated foods. If you don't eat these special foods, you have to add penalty points to your daily calculation (more about this later). The list of essential foods, along with the recommended servings, serving sizes, and number of points per

THE BLOOD SUGAR BUDGET
(You're allowed 42 to 50 points a day.)

Essential Foods	Recommended Servings	Serving Size	Points per Serving
Leafy greens and nonstarchy vegetables	5 or more per day	Leafy greens: unlimited; nonstachy veg: ½ to ¾ cup	0
Fruits	2 or 3 per day	1 small whole fruit or ½ cup cut fruit or berries	1
Extra virgin olive oil	2 to 3 per day	1 tablespoon	3
Whole grains	2 per day	1 slice or 1 muffin; ½ cup cooked grain; ½ to ¾ cup dry cereal	2
Eggs	4 or 5 per week	1 egg	2
Beans	3 or 4 times per week	½ cup cooked	2
Nuts and seeds	3 or 4 times per week of each	2 tablespoons nuts; 2 teaspoons seeds	2
Dairy	2 per day	4 to 6 ounces (½ to ⅔ cup) yogurt; 1 ounce cheese; 6 to 8 ounces (¾ to 1 cup) milk	3
Lean protein	2 per day	2 to 3 ounces at lunch; 3 to 4 ounces at dinner (max 5 to 6 ounces per day)	4 per ounce

serving, are all outlined on the chart above. We want you to become aware of not just what you are eating, but also when you are eating, so be sure to also check out the sample menus on pages 128–30 to see what this way of eating means in terms of real food. (Beware: the menus are likely to make you hungry.)

Ideally, you will eat between 42 and 50 points per day. Depending on what you choose to eat on any given day, you may end up having enough points left to splurge on a treat, like a small glass of red wine. But if you've maxed out your budget at 50 points one day because you wanted to enjoy a steak for dinner, you won't have enough points left for dessert. The good news is that you get to decide how you spend your points. Say your daily meal plan puts you at 46 points at the end of dinner. That leaves you a balance of 4 points for the day. If you decide to have a glass of wine at dinner

(5 points), you end up with a total of 51 points for the day. You will either need to deduct that additional point from your next day's allowance, or forego the wine and carry those 4 points over to the next day. As long as you've eaten all of your required budget items, it doesn't hurt to be under budget. You'll simply lose more weight and improve your blood sugar (and overall health) even faster. If you start feeling deprived, it's nice to know you have those points in the bank.

Your goal with the Blood Sugar Budget is to make smart meal and snack choices that add up to no less than 42 and no more than 50 points per day. If you've eaten all the foods required and come in under the 350 weekly point level, that's great. Keep up the good work! On a day when your points add up to a number in the low 40s, you can splurge on a potato or a small serving of pasta, or you might just eat a third piece of fruit and enjoy the extra weight loss. And your points reset every day; you wake up each morning with another 50 points to spend on healthy, healing foods.

What happens if you binge and blow it? If you're only a few points over the maximum of 50 for one day, just try to compensate by adjusting the choices you make the next day. If you went way over and dug into one of the taboo foods (see page 124), don't be too hard on yourself. Just put it out of your mind, and set your attention on getting back on track going forward. What's really important is the weekly average of 350 points, because it's what you do most of the time that counts.

At first, this new way of eating may seem like a bit of work, but keep in mind that you are retraining your dietary habits and learning how to eat correctly for diabetes control—perhaps for the first time in your life. Once you get used to using the chart to plan your meals and tally up your points, it'll become second nature. And you'll have the added pleasure of a lower A1C and a smaller waistline in just a couple of months. To see what foods fall within each category, see the lists starting on the opposite page.

LEAFY GREENS AND NONSTARCHY VEGETABLES

Artichokes
Arugula
Asparagus
Beets, raw
Bok choy
Broccoli
Brussels sprouts
Cabbage
Carrots, raw
Cauliflower
Celeriac
Collards

Cucumber
Eggplant
Fennel
Garlic
Green beans
Jerusalem artichoke
Jicama
Kale
Kohlrabi
Leeks
Lettuce

Mache
Mushrooms
Mustard greens
Okra
Onions
Parsnips
Peppers, bell
Peppers, chile
Radicchio
Radishes
Scallions
Seaweed

Shallots
Spinach
Sprouts
Summer squash
Swiss chard
Tatsoi
Tomatoes
Turnip greens
Turnips
Watercress
Zucchini

FRUITS

Apple
Apricot
Avocado
Banana
Blackberries
Blueberries
Cantaloupe

Cherries
Clementines or Mandarin oranges
Figs
Grapefruit, pink
Grapes

Kumquats
Lychees
Mango
Melon
Nectarine
Orange
Papaya

Peach
Pear
Plum
Pluot
Raspberries
Strawberries
Watermelon

WHOLE GRAINS

Amaranth
Brown rice

Buckwheat groats (kasha)
Cornmeal

Farro
Millet
Oatmeal

Quinoa
Wheat berries

BEANS

Black beans	Cranberry beans	Great Northern white beans	Pink beans
Cannellini beans	Fava beans		Pinto beans
Chickpeas (garbanzo beans)	Flageolets	Lentils	Red beans
		Navy beans	

NUTS AND SEEDS

Almonds	Pine nuts	Caraway seeds	Sesame seeds
Cashews	Pistachios	Chia seeds	Sunflower seeds
Peanuts	Walnuts	Flax seeds	
Pecans		Pumpkin seeds	

DAIRY AND DAIRY SUBSTITUTES

Almond milk (provides a good source of calcium, but contains almost no protein; keep this in mind when planning meals)

Cheese, preferably sheep's or goat's milk cheese

Soy milk, preferably fortified organic

Yogurt, preferably sheep's or goat's milk yogurt

LEAN PROTEIN

Beans (if combined with grain)	Clams	Lamb	Shrimp
	Cornish game hen	Oysters	Soy, tofu, and tempeh
Beef	Fish	Pork	Turkey
Chicken		Scallops	

FOODS TO EAT WITHIN LIMITS

In addition to all the healthful foods you must include in your diet, there are some foods, such as potatoes and winter squash, that are nutritious but contain too much starch or sugar to eat every day if you have elevated blood glucose. Likewise, semolina pasta and white rice have a higher glycemic load than many whole grains, even though they also contain valuable protein and offer tremendous gustatory pleasure. Since it's what you do most of the time that counts, you can enjoy these types of foods occasionally in limited amounts. Assume each costs 5 points and adjust your budget accordingly.

Saturated Fats

One advantage of fats is that they do not raise blood sugar. On the other hand, they are packed with calories that contribute to weight gain, and they may raise your LDL cholesterol. So while monounsaturated extra virgin olive oil is our fat of choice, a tablespoon or two of butter or sour cream no more than once a week in addition to your daily olive oil is okay. Measure carefully; do not just eyeball the amount.

Foods to Limit	Serving Size	Points per Serving
Butter	1 tablespoon	5
Mayonnaise, cream cheese, sour cream	2 tablespoons	5

Starchy and Sugary Vegetables

All vegetables are good for you, but some—such as potatoes and peas—contain so much carbohydrate (in the form of either starch or sugar) that they raise blood sugar and may contribute to weight gain. You don't need to avoid them completely; you just need to be aware of portion control and enjoy them a little less often. Potatoes, especially organic ones with their skins on, are a great source of fiber and potassium along with healthy doses of iron and vitamin C. Peas are high in protein. Beets and carrots—both rich in valuable vitamins, minerals, and antioxidants as well as fiber—are unusual in that they are relatively high in sugar, but that sugar is not always readily obtained. The tough fiber in a raw beet or carrot slows down the absorption of the sugar so much that we put it in the nonstarchy category. But cooking breaks down the fibers and makes that sugar much more likely to spike blood sugar, so cooked beets and carrots should not be eaten as often.

The glycemic load of these vegetables depends partly on their variety and how they are cooked. Steamed or boiled, waxy potatoes like Yukon golds have a relatively low glycemic load. Mashed russet potatoes, on the other hand, are similar to white bread in terms of available starch and should be eaten less often. Our advice: Eat a variety of these vegetables that are more likely to raise blood sugar no more than two or three times a week.

Foods to Limit	Serving Size	Points per Serving
Corn, peas, winter squash, potatoes, sweet potatoes, cooked beets, cooked carrots	4 to 6 ounces; ½ to ¾ cup cut vegetables	5

White Rice and Pasta

These refined carbohydrates will raise blood sugar and pack on the pounds. If you indulge, be sure it is no more than once a week in place of a whole grain. A few tips:

- Buy imported semolina pasta and cook it until al dente, just barely tender; when cooked this way, less of the carbohydrate is accessible.

- Mix cooked pasta with an equal amount of vegetables and mushrooms to balance out the carbs.

- Pair white rice, which cooks faster than brown rice and is preferred in some dishes, with beans or other vegetables. The beans and vegetables provide more fiber and balance out the carbs.

Foods to Limit	Serving Size	Points per Serving
Pasta	2 ounces (uncooked)	5
White rice	½ cup (cooked)	5

Alcohol

While very moderate alcohol consumption is sometimes associated with good health, few people who drink limit themselves to just one glass. And alcohol is high in calories and raises blood sugar. Of all the foods you can give up without harming your health, alcohol is right near the top. But since stress reduction is an important part of our program and we want this program to be realistic and achievable, we allow one glass of red wine—the healthiest of the alcohols—one or two times a week with a meal. If you only drink white wine, we'll let that go. But beer is too high in carbohydrates and hard liquor has the highest alcohol content and no nutritive value. Alcohol calories are dense: 7 calories per gram. If you're serious about losing weigh, alcohol should be the first thing you give up.

Foods to Limit	Serving Size	Points per Serving
Red wine	5 ounces	5

Dried Fruit

Raisins, dried apricots, dates, figs, and prunes are good sources of iron and they provide quick energy, but that's because they are loaded with sugar. Limit your dried fruit consumption to two or three times a week and pair them with a high-fiber food such as cereal or oatmeal, or some fat or protein like yogurt or cheese, to modulate the impact on your blood sugar.

Foods to Limit	Serving Size	Points per Serving
Raisins, dried apricots, dates, and prunes	1 to 2 tablespoons raisins; 2 or 3 dried apricots, dates, or prunes	5

EXCEPTIONS TO THE RULES

When eating in a healthy way to manage your blood sugar and gradually lose weight, it's helpful to keep in mind that rules don't have to be all or nothing.

Heavy Cream or Half-and-Half

You may have up to 1 teaspoon of heavy cream or 2 teaspoons of half-and-half in a cup of morning coffee every day for free. This adds 2 grams of fat, of which a little more than half is saturated fat. If you have more than this, add 6 points per tablespoon to your total for the day.

Sugar

You may have up to 1 teaspoon of unrefined sugar in a cup of coffee every day for free as long as you are drinking it with food. Beyond this, add 6 points per tablespoon of sugar consumed. Please avoid artificial sweeteners. Gradually train your sweet tooth to need less sugar by reducing the amount you use a little bit every couple of days. You'll be surprised at how rapidly your tastes will change.

Dark Chocolate

Two or three times a week, you can have a small square of dark chocolate (containing 72 percent cacao or more). If you eat more than this, add 4 points per ½ ounce (or tablespoon of melted chocolate).

Flour, Cornstarch, and Bread Crumbs

You may add 1 or 2 tablespoons of flour or 1 teaspoon of cornstarch to a soup or sauce to thicken it for free. Beyond this, add 2 points per every tablespoon of flour or cornstarch consumed. You may also add 2 tablespoons of bread crumbs to coat a piece of meat or top a casserole for free. After that, add 1 point per tablespoon of bread crumbs consumed.

TABOO FOODS

Some foods lack so much nutritional benefits or are so detrimental to your health that they should be avoided . . . period. Eliminate these foods from your diet completely, or if that feels impossible right now, eat them as seldom as possible and do whatever you can to cut them out gradually. These foods may be dangerous and are, most likely, habitual, so it will take some effort to avoid them, because as you'll find, eating well is a habit. The best way to stay on track is to avoid bringing these temptations into your home in the first place. If you cannot resist and you find yourself eating one of these taboo foods, it's not the end of the world. But do try to avoid making the same mistake twice—and add 8 penalty points to your day's total per serving.

Processed Meats and Fatty Cuts

Luncheon meats, ham, salami, sausages, bacon, pork belly, short ribs, beef chuck, and so on.

Not only are processed meats packed with fat, but they are also treated with nitrates and nitrites to preserve their pink color. During cooking and digestion, the nitrates and nitrites can turn into cancer-causing chemicals. We realize that these familiar foods are hard to give up, and some people recommend eating fat because it doesn't boost blood sugar, but the health detriments and cost to your waistline from eating these foods are not worth it. When you absolutely need a fix, look for a nitrate-free or "uncured" product.

Refined Carbohydrates

Foods made with white flour and added sugar, such as white bread, bagels, biscuits, chips, muffins, cakes, pies, cookies, ice cream, frozen desserts, and so on.

If you're honest with yourself, you know these are the foods that pack on the pounds. And in recent years, we've learned that these refined carbohydrates contribute as much or more to raising LDL cholesterol than saturated fat. In terms of blood sugar levels, these carbs are just many, many sugar molecules all strung together. Keep these out of your home, and try to find a substitute whenever you can: a whole-grain equivalent, fruit and cheese, fruit and nuts, or a small square of dark chocolate. The reason sweets and crisp, salty snacks are so difficult to give up is because they are addicting. You'll find that if you forego these blood sugar busters for a few days, you will quickly begin to crave them less.

Note: We've included some dessert recipes (see page 217) for special occasions. These dishes pair sugar with nuts, fruit, and cream to minimize the damage the sugar can cause. These desserts also are served in very small portions and designed to be eaten strictly after a meal. We've added up the points of the dessert recipes for you, but when you're making your own desserts, add 6 points per tablespoon of heavy cream or sugar.

Fried Foods, Processed Foods, and Trans Fats

French fries, onion wings, fried chicken or fish, fried pastries and donuts, and crispy snacks like potato and tortilla chips. All foods that are precooked and chemically manipulated, such as luncheon meats and packaged foods. Trans fats are most commonly found in fried foods, ice cream and frozen yogurt, and such store-bought baked goods as cookies and cakes.

Fried foods are a no-no because of their fat content, potential for containing trans fats, and huge load of calories. Processed foods, especially fat-free products, should also be avoided because they are packed with food additives and carbohydrates. Many of the so-called "modified starches," such as dextrin and maltodextrin, are artificially developed either to mimic the sensation of fat in the mouth or keep food fresh. We're not sure yet what these do to your gut, but you can bet the house that chips—whether potato, corn, or pita—will pack on the pounds.

Remember when margarine was thought to be healthier than butter? Well, not anymore. We've learned that in terms of damage to our arteries, artificial trans fats are at the top of the list of offenders. These days, most manufacturers are trying to phase out trans fats from their products. Since a loophole in the law does not require small amounts to be listed on packages, it's best to avoid the kind of products known to contain them.

Sugar-Sweetened Beverages

Colas, other sodas, and sweet tea.

Sweetened beverages spike blood sugar levels and have been firmly linked to obesity. Many colas contain a carcinogenic chemical, and the sodas are so acidic that they can contribute to the development of osteoporosis. Find yourself a good substitute, such as a pleasant herbal tea or club soda with 1 to 2 teaspoons of fruit syrup and a squeeze of lemon or lime.

Artificial and Alternative Sweeteners

Equal, Splenda, Sweet'N Low, NutraSweet, stevia, and the like.

We greatly discourage the use of artificial sweeteners and other sugar substitutes because they have unnaturally strong sweetening power. All they do is raise your sugar bar and keep you addicted to sweets and refined carbohydrates. Studies have shown that artificial sweeteners are counterproductive to losing weight. In fact, diet sodas have been linked to obesity.

Recording what you eat and drink in detail over the course of the day will make it easy to tally the number of points you've spent each week. Many of our patients tell us that when they record what they eat, it makes them much more mindful; sometimes they are surprised at what they are (or are not) eating and in what quantities. Sticking to the Blood Sugar Budget means not only avoiding the foods with high point values, but also making sure you get enough of the foods you must eat every day. So that you don't skimp on your nutrient-rich foods, there are a few penalties that—like the taboo foods—require you to add 8 points to your daily tally:

- If you don't eat at least 5 leafy greens and nonstarchy vegetables every day
- If you don't have at least 2 servings of dairy per day
- It you don't have at least 1 serving of whole grains every day

PLANNING YOUR MEALS

When you're first starting to use the Blood Sugar Budget, it's helpful to plan out your meals ahead of time. Doing this planning on a weekly basis will help you track the number of points you're eating and ensure that you're eating all the essential foods, including the required daily servings of leafy greens and nonstarchy vegetables (at least five servings), dairy (at least two servings), and whole grains (at least one serving). Use our recipes or your own to inspire creative and varied menus, and make sure your choices add up to 50 points or less per day.

To show you a few examples of what you might eat in a day, take a look at the three menus that follow. All comply with the budget. Two are everyday menus, and one includes a weekend dinner party. Once you plan your meals a few times, you'll begin to see some patterns. You know that most vegetables are free (meaning, they don't cost any points, except when you don't eat enough of them), but in terms of filling your belly, you'll begin to realize just how wonderful salads and cooked vegetables are. You can eat a whole lot of both, and then have flexibility elsewhere for special treats or limited foods you love. Likewise, you'll begin to realize how expensive sweets, protein, and limited foods are. And before long, you'll be able to plan your meals without counting points at all.

Here's an example of a really healthy menu that gives you everything you need with little fuss. It also balances your carbohydrates throughout the day, which is best for blood sugar control.

Breakfast: 6 points (1 fruit, 1 whole grain, 1 dairy)

- 1 clementine
- ½ cup steel-cut oatmeal
- 1 cup soy milk
- Cup of coffee with 1 teaspoon heavy cream

Snack: 2 points (1 fruit, ½ nuts)

- 1 small apple
- 1 tablespoon almonds
- Cup of herbal tea

Lunch: 17 points (5 nonstarchy vegetables, 1⅓ olive oil, 1 whole grain, 1 dairy, 2 ounces lean protein)

- Turkey chef's salad: Romaine lettuce, tomato, cucumber, celery, red onion, 2 ounces roast turkey, and 1 ounce Cheddar, Manchego, or blue cheese, dressed with 1 tablespoon extra virgin olive oil, 1 teaspoon lemon juice, and 1 teaspoon red wine vinegar
- 1 slice whole grain bread, toasted, rubbed with garlic, and brushed with 1 teaspoon extra virgin olive oil
- Cup of herbal tea

Snack: 2 points (2 nonstarchy vegetables, 1 beans)

- ½ cup hummus with carrot and red bell pepper sticks

Dinner: 21 points (3 nonstarchy vegetables, 1 fruit, 1 olive oil, ½ whole grain, 4 ounces lean protein)

- Lemony Escarole and Rice Soup (page 164)
- 4 ounces broiled salmon served with lemon wedges
- 1 cup steamed broccoli drizzled with 1 teaspoon each extra virgin olive oil and lemon juice
- ⅔ cup steamed zucchini drizzled with 1 teaspoon each extra virgin olive oil and balsamic vinegar
- ½ cup cherries

This menu illustrates how combined complementary vegetable proteins can stand in for lean protein sources while giving you one of your week's bean allowances as well.

Breakfast: 9 points (1 nonstarchy vegetables, 1 fruit, 1½ eggs, ½ olive oil, 1 whole grain, ½ dairy)

- Wedge of cantaloupe
- Asparagus Frittata with Goat Cheese (page 157)
- 1 high-fiber whole grain English muffin
- Cup of coffee with 1 teaspoon heavy cream

Snack: 4 points (1 fruit, 1 dairy)

- ⅔ cup whole goat's milk yogurt with ½ cup blueberries

Lunch: 9 points (2 nonstarchy vegetables, 1 fruit, ⅓ olive oil, 1 whole grain, 1 beans, 1 dairy)

- Black Bean Taquitos (page 196)
- ½ cup diced mango
- Cup of herbal tea

Snack: 3 points (2 nonstarchy vegetables, 1 dairy)

- Cucumber Sandwiches with Goat Cheese and Arugula (page 146)
- Cup of herbal tea

Dinner: 21 points (4 nonstarchy vegetables, 1 olive oil, 1 whole grain, 4 ounces lean protein)

- Small spinach salad with grape tomatoes, shredded carrots, and sliced hearts of palm, dressed with 1 teaspoon extra virgin olive oil, 1 teaspoon fresh lemon juice, and splash of sherry vinegar
- 4 ounces rotisserie chicken (skin removed)
- Lemony Stir-Fried Brussels Sprouts (page 204)
- ½ cup cooked quinoa

Since this is a special dinner party menu, the end of the day is heavily weighted. It was tight, but we squeezed in a dinner with dessert and still kept to our budget by only allowing fruit for snacks.

Breakfast: 6 points (1 fruit, 1 whole grain, 1 dairy)

- 1 clementine
- ⅔ cup high-fiber cereal
- 1 cup soy milk
- Cup of coffee with 1 teaspoon heavy cream

Snack: 1 point (1 fruit)

- 1 small apple
- Cup of green tea

Lunch: 12 points (4 nonstarchy vegetables, 1 olive oil, ½ beans, 2 ounces lean protein)

- Arugula with tomatoes, red bell peppers, and radishes, dressed with 1 tablespoon extra virgin olive oil, 1 teaspoon lemon juice, and 1 teaspoon white wine vinegar
- ½ can tuna (about 2 ounces)
- ¼ cup chickpeas
- Cup of herbal tea

Snack: 3 points (1 nonstarchy vegetables, 1 dairy)

- Carrot sticks and 1 ounce Manchego cheese
- Cup of herbal tea

Dinner Party: 28 points (4 nonstarchy vegetables, 1 fruit, 1 olive oil, 1 whole grain, ½ egg, 1 nuts, ⅔ dairy, 3 ounces lean protein, about 1 sugar)

- Chilled Avocado and Cucumber Soup (made with soy milk; page 164)
- 3 ounces filet mignon (grilled rare)
- Slow-roasted tomatoes, steamed green beans, and steamed or roasted cauliflower drizzled with 1 tablespoon extra virgin olive oil and 2 teaspoons balsamic vinegar
- ½ cup wild rice
- Hazelnut Torte (page 220) with a small drizzle of melted bittersweet chocolate

HOW YOU SHOULD EAT

Whew, that was a lot of information to absorb. But since repetition never hurts, here are some more tips for following the Blood Sugar Budget.

- Never skip meals.
- Try to eat at the same time every day.
- Strive for three smaller meals and a couple of healthy snacks. Carbohydrates should be distributed evenly throughout the day. Portion control is vital, so be sure to follow the recommended serving sizes.
- Eat a high-fiber diet. This means eating cereal with at least 5 grams of fiber per serving (follow our recommended serving sizes or check the label); whole grain rather than white bread; modest amounts of nuts, seeds, and beans; lots of vegetables; and two fruits a day.
- Avoid sugar, sweet desserts, and artificial sweeteners. If you do have a starch or carbohydrate, like bread or crackers, try to pair it with some protein or a healthy fat like a small amount of peanut butter or a slice of cheese; partner fruit with cheese or yogurt.
- Two-thirds of your plate should consist of vegetables of different colors. Add to that a small serving (½ cup) of a whole grain such as quinoa or rice or a small amount of potatoes (not fried). Lean protein such as fish, chicken, or turkey completes the plate. (Tofu and beans are also good sources of lean protein, but the beans must be paired with a grain to give you all the nutrition you need.)
- When eating red meat, which includes beef, pork, and lamb, choose lean cuts, trim off any excess fat, and check your portion size. Just 2 to 3 ounces for lunch and 3 to 4 ounces for dinner will give you what you need.
- Indulge in healthy oils, especially extra virgin olive oil, which has proven anti-inflammatory and protective benefits. You should have 2 to 3 tablespoons a day, with about half of that uncooked (used in dressing for a salad, for instance).
- Eat small amounts of whole- or reduced-fat dairy products, especially yogurt and cheese. Avoid low-fat and nonfat dairy products. This may sound counterintuitive to weight loss, but the full-fat products are better for blood sugar control, and the difference in calories in modest portions is not great.

Leafy Greens and Nonstarchy Vegetables (5 or more servings per day)

Vegetables are a major part of the Blood Sugar Budget. The easiest way to get all the vegetables you need is to have a salad and two cooked vegetables every day—it's that simple. Your salad can be a small side salad before or with dinner, or it could be a main course salad for lunch, loaded with goodies. But it must have at least three vegetables, preferably of different colors, which indicate different phytochemicals—plant compounds that may protect our health and reduce the risk of some chronic diseases. One of those could be raw spinach, which would satisfy your requirement for at least one leafy green per day, or it could be many lettuces you like, along with at least two other vegetables—raw or leftover cooked.

You can lightly steam almost any vegetable in about 3 minutes, so it's an easy and efficient way to get your vegetables. Or you can toss them in olive oil and roast them. Dress raw and lightly steamed greens with a teaspoon of fresh lemon juice and two teaspoons of extra virgin olive oil in addition to a splash of your favorite vinegar, if you wish. The lemon juice helps you absorb the minerals from your vegetables. Any time you prefer to make a more complex preparation, of course you can. Aim for a variety of vegetables over the week, and make sure that one of your vegetables, either raw or cooked, is a leafy dark green: spinach, chard, kale, broccoli, collards, or brussels sprouts, for example. Many people who used to think they didn't like brussels sprouts have changed their minds now that they've learned how to roast them.

These should be the mainstay of your diet. Whenever you have a dish that is not a vegetable, like a sandwich instead of a salad or steamed vegetables, ask yourself, "Where are my veggies?" Carrot sticks, tomatoes, cucumbers, radishes, bell pepper strips, even a few sweet potato chips, can accompany a sandwich. Nonstarchy vegetables like tomatoes, raw carrots, broccoli, asparagus, zucchini, greens (turnip, collards, kale, spinach, and so on), and other vegetables are full of fiber, vitamins, and such minerals as calcium, potassium, and magnesium. Consider these vegetables free. They will fill you up with healthy fiber, vitamins, minerals, and antioxidants at a cost of very few calories.

LEAFY GREEN VEGETABLES

Leafy greens such as lettuce, spinach, cabbage, collards, kale, chard, arugula, broccoli, and brussels sprouts are richly nutritious and high in fiber. In general, the darker the green, the more vitamins and minerals you'll receive. All of these vegetables contain folate, a B vitamin that's important for everyone but especially for women in their childbearing years. Leafy greens also contain calcium, magnesium, iron, vitamin A, vitamin C, vitamin E, and short-chain fatty acids that are converted into vitamin K in the gut and are essential for blood clotting and bone health. Keep in mind, especially if you prefer a more plant-based diet, that almost any serving of a vegetable contains 2 or 3 grams of protein. Although by itself a vegetable does not contain all the essential amino acids you need for growth and healing, its protein can combine with meat, cheese, or eggs or with complementary grains and legumes to add to your protein stores.

The nutrients in vegetables are a little harder to absorb than those in meat, but they are highly beneficial because they contain no saturated fat and are very low in calories. So to help your body absorb the nutrients from these vegetables, whether raw or lightly steamed, dress them with a modest amount of extra virgin olive oil and a teaspoon or two of freshly squeezed lemon juice. You can also splash on your favorite vinegar for added flavor.

Fruits (2 or 3 servings per day)

Although they don't contribute protein to your diet, fruits are rich in fiber, potassium, and magnesium, and usually low in fat. Examples of a serving include 1 small whole fruit or ½ cup cut-up fruit or berries. Pineapples are high in carbohydrates, so keep these amounts smaller. One whole banana or avocado is worth 2 points (or 1 point per half).

Extra Virgin Olive Oil (2 to 3 tablespoons per day)

Fat helps your body absorb essential vitamins and bolsters your immune system. While saturated fat and trans fat have been implicated in cardio-vascular disease, monounsaturated fat—especially extra virgin olive oil—has been shown to have tremendous protective benefits. Large studies have associated this healthy oil with a lower risk of many chronic diseases, including diabetes, heart disease, and high blood pressure.

Whole Grains (2 servings per day)

There's a tendency these days to avoid grains, but studies have shown that they are helpful with glycemic control. Examples of one serving of grains include a slice of whole grain bread, a high-fiber muffin, ½ to ¾ cup dry cereal, or ½ cup cooked grain. Read labels because some whole wheat products contain too much sweetener to be helpful.

Eggs (4 or 5 eggs per week)

Eating the recommended number of eggs each week is an important part of a healthy diet. And when we say egg, we're talking about the whole egg: the white and the yolk. Complete protein is distributed throughout the egg, but it's the yolk that contains all the iron, biotin, choline, and vitamins A, D, B_6, and B_{12}. Some of these nutrients are hard to find elsewhere, especially for people who don't eat much meat. While eggs were maligned for some years, we now recognize that dietary cholesterol is rarely the problem we thought it was, and a certain amount of cholesterol is vital for the health of your cell walls and production of sex hormones. That said, it is recommended you don't eat more than two eggs at a single meal.

Beans (3 or 4 servings per week)

Beans and other legumes like lentils and chickpeas are fabulous foods for lowering blood sugar. While beans do contain carbohydrates, they are very high in protein, rich in fiber, and good sources of folate, potassium, calcium, and iron. Regular consumption of beans in a healthy diet has been shown to lower blood sugar and blood pressure, and is associated with less type 2 diabetes and lower weight. That said, portion size matters (as with all foods). In the Blood Sugar Budget, the serving size of ½ cup is for beans eaten as a side dish, which you might enjoy a few days a week. You can also toss ¼ cup of beans (a half serving) onto a salad any day; in that case, only charge yourself 1 point (or half the number of points per serving). You might also use beans as your lean protein source—such as in a vegetarian chili—once or twice a week. In this case, you can allow yourself a double portion of beans (1 cup), which would count as 4 points. If you

Drinking enough fluids every day is important for healthy eating. You need 8 to 10 cups, or 2 to 2½ liters, of liquid per day to optimize your bodily functions and keep your blood properly hydrated. As an added benefit, the fluids you need for your health will also help fill you up, so keeping hydrated functions as a weight loss aide, too. Water is the number one choice for staying hydrated, but coffee, herbal tea, and soup all count. Fruit juice contains too much sugar and calories to be a good choice. And, no surprise, sodas and sweet tea are off limits, whether they are sweetened with sugar or artificial sweeteners.

You might think drinking enough water would be a no-brainer, but we don't always feel thirsty. In fact, as we age, the sensation of thirst diminishes. If you're over the age of seventy or you know that you're one of the many people who don't drink enough water, it's a good idea to set up a system to help you stay hydrated. There are several options: Create a task on your tablet or smart phone to remind you to drink a glass of water a few times per day, fill a 2-liter thermos with your favorite healthy beverage and commit to drinking the whole thing by the end of the day, or use a hydration cup to keep track of the number of cups you have downed.

are eating beans as a meat substitute, keep in mind that legumes are not a complete protein. They lack one essential amino acid, methionine. That's why when beans are eaten as a vegetarian alternative, they must be paired with a grain, such as rice, corn, or wheat. (Soybean-based products, such as tofu and tempeh, are good alternatives to meat because they contain all of the amino acids your body needs to make a complete protein.)

Nuts and Seeds (3 or 4 servings per week of each)

These contribute protein, fiber, healthy oils, B vitamins, and minerals to your diet. The serving size (2 tablespoons of nuts and 2 teaspoons of seeds) is small because these foods are high in calories. Nuts in small amounts make a good snack, especially when paired with a small piece of fruit. Almonds, in particular, are rich in calcium. Seeds can be sprinkled over cereal or salads.

Dairy (2 servings per day)

Yogurt, cheese, and other dairy products are major sources of calcium, vitamin D, and protein. We prefer that you have yogurt or sheep's milk or goat's milk cheese as your protein source, along with fortified, organic soy milk. Cow's milk is high in sugar and carbohydrates and it is a very inflammatory food; other sources of calcium are preferable. While most diets, including the American version of the Mediterranean Diet, call for low-fat dairy, the truth is that in the Mediterranean countries where dietary patterns have been equated with better health—including lower risk of diabetes, cardiovascular disease, and even cancer—adults do not drink milk. They do eat modest amounts of full-fat yogurt and artisanal cheeses, usually made from sheep's or goat's milk. As mentioned elsewhere in this book, recent studies have associated some saturated dairy fats with better glycemic control and lower blood sugar. That's why we recommend measured amounts of full-fat yogurt and cheeses in the Blood Sugar Budget. That said, please keep in mind that cream cheese and ice cream should be considered occasional treats, not healthy dairy.

Lean Protein (5 to 6 ounces per day)

Meat can be a rich source of protein, B vitamins, iron, and zinc. But for reasons not yet fully understood, consumption of red meat is not associated with good health statistically, so don't make it a mainstay of your diet. We recommend eating red meat—beef, pork, or lamb—no more than once a week. Cut back on your typical meat portions by one-third or one-half and pile on the vegetables instead. Examples of one serving include 2 to 3 ounces of cooked skinless poultry or lean meat, 3 to 4 ounces of fish, 1 egg, or 2 ounces (half a can) of light—not white—tuna, or salmon or sardines, preferably with the bones.

Eat heart-healthy fish, such as salmon, herring, and tuna. These types of fish are high in omega-3 fatty acids, which contribute to better health in many ways because they are anti-inflammatory. If you don't eat fish, be sure to take pharmaceutical-grade fish oil pills. Trim away skin and fat from meat and poultry, then broil, grill, roast, or poach instead of frying.

Why Breakfast Is Important

Many people think they cannot tolerate putting anything in their mouth when they first get up, except perhaps a cup of coffee. Learning to eat a nutritious breakfast is a challenge for many people. But just like exercise, once you get into it, you'll find you miss it if you stop. And it's extremely important for proper glucose control. Many people think that if they don't eat or they skip a meal, they'll keep their blood sugar as low as possible and avoid insulin spikes. But the truth is, if you don't eat, your body still needs more fuel than it can get from breaking down fat. So your liver (which also produces glucose) will start pumping it out on the spot, defeating your entire purpose of skipping a meal. A number of studies have associated eating a substantial breakfast with better weight control as well as better performance in school for children.

Because the liver produces sugar overnight, when you are inadvertently fasting, blood glucose levels tend to be a little higher in the morning. Because of this, breakfast should be a little lower in carbohydrates than other meals, but morning offers a good opportunity to enjoy an egg, a small amount of oatmeal or high-fiber cold cereal, yogurt with a little fruit and some muesli or lower-calorie granola, or a single slice of whole grain toast with some cheese. Fruit in moderation is not amiss, with perhaps half a pink grapefruit (if you're not on statins) or some berries or a small apple along with coffee or tea.

SWEETS

You don't have to banish sweets entirely; just go easy on them. Use ½ cup of sorbet or frozen yogurt as a reward for following the Blood Sugar Budget the rest of the week. However, when you do eat sweets, make sure you're not eating them on an empty stomach; they are best eaten after a full meal.

Note: Cut back on added sugar, which has no nutritional value but can pack on the calories. Artificial sweeteners such as aspartame (NutraSweet, Equal), sucralose (Splenda), and saccharin (Sweet'N Low) may help satisfy your sweet tooth while sparing the calories, but these ingredients have been associated with obesity in many studies, and we do not recommend them. Some integrative nutritionists worry about their long-term health effects, as well. Even though no harm has been proven in humans, some animal studies have been disturbing.

THE BLOOD SUGAR BUDGET RECIPES

Because you're not always going to eat single foods—an apple, a grilled chicken breast—and because eating a variety of delicious dishes is the best incentive for changing your eating habits, our one hundred recipes combine all of the essential foods we recommend, along with some of the foods we want you to limit. And each recipe lists the total point value per serving (when in doubt, we've rounded up).

As you'll see in chapter 9, many of these dishes cost very little in terms of the Blood Sugar Budget. That's because when you eat foods that are best for controlling your diabetes—and for maintaining good health in general—there's plenty of room for good eating without deprivation. Excessive protein (especially in the form of red meat), saturated fats, fried foods, and starches are the categories that get expensive. We hope you'll see how you can avoid these foods and instead turn to healthy vegetables, fruits, and appropriate dairy.

It's also important to eat mixed foods. That means pair a carbohydrate like fruit with some protein and/or fat, such as a small piece of cheese or a few nuts. The protein and fat, which take longer to digest, and the fiber from whole grains, fruits, and vegetables, slow the passage of food through the gut and modulate the absorption of glucose. That's why many of our mixed dishes are rich in dietary fiber.

In addition, we encourage anyone who values their health to eat organic as much as possible, and read nutrition labels so you know what you're putting inside your body.

We've designed over one hundred recipes to benefit your health by being low in glycemic index or glycemic load (see page 108) and rich in fiber. And to make it simple, we tag each recipe with the appropriate number of points, so you know how much of a bite it's taking out of your budget. Many of these will be a pleasant surprise. You get a lot of food and flavor for little cost. Some are low or moderate in calories; all except a few desserts are also low in refined carbohydrates. You don't need to use these recipes, but they are tasty and fit easily into the Blood Sugar Budget. Even just reading over them and seeing what they cost in budget points will give you a better idea of which foods you can afford.

Simple whole foods are good for you, but an apple, a stick of celery, and a broiled chicken breast are not what you are going to be happy eating all the time. So these diabetes-friendly recipes offer wide variety.

WHY THE BLOOD SUGAR BUDGET WORKS

Choosing your foods according to the guidelines set out in the Blood Sugar Budget will reduce elevated glucose levels because it:

- Encourages weight loss. Remember, losing just 5 to 7 percent of your current body weight usually achieves lower blood sugar, lower blood pressure, and often better cholesterol levels.

- Feeds the good bacteria in your gut. These microscopic organisms help us digest our food, metabolize nutrients, stimulate insulin production, strengthen the immune system, and help break down fat.

- Reduces inflammation. Type 2 diabetes is an inflammatory disease, and many of the foods you must eat on the Blood Sugar Budget, such as olive oil and leafy green vegetables, are anti-inflammatory.

If you stay on budget for as little as ten days, you'll be surprised by how fast you start feeling lighter and more energetic, focused, and relaxed. After as little as a month or two, you should see improvements in both your weight and your A1C. We can't wait to hear about your success on the Blood Sugar Budget.

THE RECIPES

APPETIZERS AND SNACKS

Appetizers can make meals more interesting and actually help you eat less. That's because it takes about twenty minutes for your satiety hormones to kick in. So if you have a small appetizer to begin with, by the time you get to the main course, you won't be as hungry and will be satisfied with a smaller portion. At the same time, a first course can make mealtime more entertaining. These same foods often double as snacks, which are very helpful for keeping blood sugar even between meals. By fending off extreme hunger, especially in the late afternoon, they prevent bingeing after work and before dinner, when many people are ravenous and grab whatever is at hand.

Aioli (aka Garlic Mayonnaise) with Spring Vegetables

8 SERVINGS | 6 POINTS EACH

Aioli is both the name of the dish and the garlic mayonnaise that is its signature. Choose your vegetables for a variety of colors and textures. You can include some small boiled potatoes and even poached fish, if you like.

3 or 4 cloves garlic	1 farm-fresh egg yolk	Pinch of raw sugar
½ teaspoon sea salt or coarse kosher salt	3 to 4 teaspoons freshly squeezed lemon juice	Assortment of raw or lightly steamed vegetables, chosen for color and texture
1 cup fruity extra-virgin olive oil	2 teaspoons water	
	½ teaspoon Dijon mustard	

In a marble or stone mortar and pestle, pound the garlic with the salt to form a paste. Gradually work in 2 tablespoons of the olive oil until you have a fairly smooth, almost fluffy puree.

Briefly whirl the egg yolk in a food processor. Add the garlic puree and, with the machine on, gradually add 2 more tablespoons of the olive oil through the feed tube. Continue to process, gradually adding 2 teaspoons of the lemon juice and the water, then slowly drizzle in the remaining ¾ cup oil. Don't worry if a bit of the oil remains puddled around the blade.

Scrape the aioli into a small bowl, using a scraper to get all the oil out of the machine. Whisk in the mustard, sugar, and the remaining 1 to 2 teaspoons of lemon juice if you'd like. Season with additional salt to taste. If not using at once, cover and refrigerate for up to 3 days.

To serve, arrange the vegetables on a platter. Pass the bowl of aioli on the side.

Zesty Kale Dip

MAKES ¾ CUP; 4 SERVINGS | 2 POINTS EACH

A creamy, flavorful dip surrounded by a colorful assortment of crisp vegetables is always a hit at parties. Should you be lucky enough to have any left over, a mere spoonful will add pizzazz to a plain grilled chicken breast.

1½ cups (packed) coarsely chopped fresh kale leaves (stems and tough central rib removed)

1 scallion, coarsely chopped

2 tablespoons freshly grated Parmesan cheese

2 tablespoons extra-virgin olive oil

1 clove garlic, coarsely chopped

⅛ teaspoon salt

6 ounces (about ⅔ cup) plain whole-milk yogurt, preferably goat's milk yogurt

---

In a food processor or blender, combine the kale, scallion, Parmesan, oil, garlic, and salt. Pulse the machine on and off until the kale is very finely chopped.

Add the yogurt and process until well blended. Transfer to a bowl and serve at once, or cover and refrigerate for up to 24 hours.

Hot Garlic and Anchovy Dip with Assorted Vegetables

6 SERVINGS | 7 POINTS EACH

This is what Italians call *bagna cauda*, or hot pot. Although it looks like a lot of oil, very little of it actually clings, and most of the fat is healthy extra-virgin olive oil. If you enjoy spicy heat, add a pinch of crushed hot red pepper.

⅔ cup fruity extra-virgin olive oil

1½ tablespoons unsalted butter

4 cloves garlic, finely chopped

1 ounce flat anchovy fillets, chopped

Salt and freshly ground pepper

3 or 4 cups prepared raw vegetables: cherry or grape tomatoes, Belgian endive spears, bell pepper strips, radishes (halved lengthwise if large), carrot sticks, cut-up raw fennel or celery, cauliflower florets, lightly steamed asparagus or broccoli, blanched snow peas or sugar snap peas

---

In a small saucepan or fondue pot, heat the oil. Add the butter, garlic, and anchovies. Cook over medium-low heat, stirring often, until the garlic is soft and the anchovies have dissolved, about 3 minutes.

Season lightly with salt and generously with freshly ground pepper. Serve as a warm dipping sauce for the vegetables.

Cucumber Sandwiches
with Goat Cheese and Arugula

MAKES 8 SANDWICHES; 4 SERVINGS | 2 POINTS EACH

At about 15 calories each, these tasty little hors d'oeuvres let you indulge a bit. They work as well at a cocktail party as they do as a mid-morning or an afternoon snack, or as an added component to a salad plate. They are best freshly made because then they are pleasingly crisp. A tiny bit of smoked salmon would not be amiss. If you don't have arugula, watercress or dill is a good substitute. This recipe makes 8 tiny "sandwiches"; double it exactly for 16.

½ seedless English cucumber	1 tablespoon full-fat sour cream	1 teaspoon finely minced shallot
2 ounces fresh white goat cheese (chèvre)	¼ cup coarsely chopped arugula	Salt and freshly ground pepper

Peel the cucumber lengthwise in strips at intervals to create green and white stripes. On a slight angle, cut into at least 16 slices, about ¼ inch thick.

In a small bowl, blend together the goat cheese and sour cream until smooth. Stir in the arugula and shallot. Season with salt and pepper to taste.

Spread 1½ to 2 teaspoons of the goat cheese mixture over each of 8 cucumber slices. Top with the other slices to make little sandwiches. Press lightly to help them hold together. Eat at once or wrap well and refrigerate for up to a day.

Cheesy Brussels Bites

6 SERVINGS | 2 POINTS EACH

Who would have believed that brussels sprouts would become the new "it" vegetable? They are wonderful prepared many ways. This savory preparation is designed as a pick-up hors d'oeuvre or snack, but you could also eat them as a side dish.

1 pound brussels sprouts, preferably small or medium	2 teaspoons sea salt	6 tablespoons finely grated Parmigiano-Reggiano cheese
2 tablespoons extra-virgin olive oil	2 teaspoons turbinado or demerara sugar	

Preheat the oven to 375°F. Trim the stem ends from the brussels sprouts and cut any large ones in half.

In a bowl, toss the brussels sprouts with the oil, salt, and sugar. Arrange on a baking sheet in a single layer and roast until tender and lightly browned in spots, 25 to 30 minutes. Let cool slightly.

Raise the oven temperature to 400°F. Return the sprouts to the bowl and toss with the grated cheese to coat. Arrange again on the baking sheet and roast until the cheese just melts, 3 to 5 minutes.

Serve warm or at room temperature. Eat with toothpicks or your fingers.

Roasted Eggplant and Walnut Dip

MAKES ABOUT 1½ CUPS; 6 SERVINGS | 2 POINTS EACH

Eggplant is meaty and satisfying and has a very low glycemic index (see page 108). This classic Greek dip blends the roasted vegetable with walnuts, garlic, and parsley. Though the pomegranate seeds are optional, include them if you can; they are not only pretty but also full of antioxidants. Serve as an appetizer with carrot sticks, Belgian endive spears, or a few pita triangles. Or spread on rye crisps for a light snack. This recipe doubles easily for a party.

1 large Italian eggplant (about 1½ pounds)	2 tablespoons extra-virgin olive oil	Salt and freshly ground pepper
⅓ cup parsley leaves	1 tablespoon freshly squeezed lemon juice	⅓ cup fresh pomegranate seeds (optional)
¼ cup walnut pieces	2 teaspoons pomegranate molasses	
1 clove garlic, crushed		

Preheat the oven to 425°F. Pierce the eggplant in a few places and place on a baking sheet. Roast for 45 to 55 minutes, turning once or twice, until the eggplant is slightly blackened and deflated. Remove and let cool slightly.

As soon as the eggplant is cool enough to handle, cut it in half and scoop out the softened flesh into a food processor. Add any juices that accumulate on the cutting board to the processor. Add the parsley, walnuts, garlic, oil, lemon juice, and pomegranate molasses. Process until coarsely pureed. Season with salt and pepper to taste.

Transfer to a serving bowl. Stir in the pomegranate seeds. Cover and refrigerate until serving time.

Hunan Chicken Lettuce Roll-Ups

4 SERVINGS | 10 POINTS EACH

This Asian-inspired finger food serves equally well as a light lunch.

6 dried shiitake mushrooms	½ cup finely diced water chestnuts	1 tablespoon hoisin sauce
12 ounces small skinless, boneless chicken breasts	2 scallions, chopped	2 teaspoons soy sauce
	2 tablespoons chopped cilantro	1 teaspoon sesame oil
		12 butter lettuce or inner romaine leaves

Soak the mushrooms in hot water until soft, about 15 minutes. Lift out and squeeze excess water back into the bowl. Remove the stems and chop into fine dice.

In a small saucepan of simmering salted water, poach the chicken over medium-low heat until just cooked through but still moist, 7 to 9 minutes. Remove the chicken and let cool slightly. Chop into fine dice.

In a bowl, combine the diced chicken, mushrooms, water chestnuts, scallions, cilantro, hoisin sauce, soy sauce, and sesame oil. Toss to mix well.

Put about 2 tablespoons of filling in the center of each lettuce leaf and roll it up like a cigar. Eat with your fingers.

Peanut Butter-Sweet Potato Dip

MAKES ABOUT 1½ CUPS; 6 SERVINGS | 3 POINTS EACH

Snacking is something of an art. It's helpful for keeping blood sugar levels even and reducing hunger so you don't overeat at mealtime. But aside from fruits and vegetables, finding healthy foods that won't bust the calorie budget is not easy. The trick is choosing the right ingredients and exercising strict portion control. At a party, you can splurge, but for in-between meals, allow yourself ⅓ cup of this dip with ½ apple and 8 sweet potato chips for scooping.

1 sweet potato or garnet yam, 6 ounces	½ cup plain whole-milk yogurt, preferably goat's milk yogurt	Dash of Cackalacky Spice Sauce or other hot sauce
1½ tablespoons natural peanut butter		

Preheat the oven to 400°F. Put the sweet potato on a sheet of aluminum foil or in a small baking dish. Prick in 2 or 3 places and put in the oven. Roast for 40 to 45 minutes, or until very soft. Remove and let stand until cool enough to handle.

Cut the sweet potato in half lengthwise and scoop the warm flesh into a mini-processor. Add the peanut butter and blend well. (You can also do this by hand with a fork.) Add the yogurt and hot sauce and whirl until fluffy and well mixed. Serve at room temperature or slightly chilled.

Smoked Trout in Endive Spears

8 SERVINGS | 6 POINTS EACH

Trout is a light fish, whether smoked or not. A mild horseradish cream blended with fresh herbs binds the fish into a delicate salad served on Belgian endive spears. For a party, try to find a mix of red and white endive, and arrange the spears in a sunflower pattern on a large round platter.

3 tablespoons full-fat sour cream	2 tablespoons drained white horseradish	2 teaspoons freshly squeezed lemon juice
3 tablespoons plain whole-milk yogurt, preferably goat's milk yogurt	1 tablespoon finely chopped dill, plus sprigs for garnish	Salt and freshly ground pepper
	2 teaspoons minced shallot	6 ounces smoked trout
		2 heads Belgian endive

In a small bowl, blend together the sour cream and yogurt. Stir in the horseradish, chopped dill, shallot, and lemon juice. Season lightly with salt and generously with pepper.

Flake the trout and add it to the horseradish cream. Stir to blend well. Dollop about 1½ teaspoons onto the wider stem end of each endive spear. Arrange attractively on a platter. Garnish each with a tiny sprig of dill.

BREAKFAST AND BRUNCH

As we've said before, skipping breakfast is no way to lose weight. On the contrary, having a well-balanced, nutritious morning meal is associated with better weight control and blood glucose control. Here you'll find a wide variety of tasty ideas. Some, such as the Egyptian Breakfast Beans (page 155) and the Smoked Turkey Hash (page 153), can even stand in for a light supper.

Breakfast Burrito

1 SERVING | 8 POINTS

Quick and tasty, this is a fine breakfast for weekday or weekend brunch. The only problem is you're going to want to eat at least two, and that would not be helpful. So before you have your burrito, enjoy your morning coffee or tea with half a pink grapefruit or a 2-inch wedge of cantaloupe.

1 (8-inch) whole wheat tortilla wrapper	Pinch of salt	1½ tablespoons shredded Cheddar, Monterey Jack, or Manchego cheese
2½ tablespoons fat-free refried beans, such as Trader Joe's brand	Dash of Tabasco sauce or your favorite hot sauce	
1 egg	1½ teaspoons extra-virgin olive oil	1 tablespoon salsa, or more to taste
		1 tablespoon chopped scallion or white onion

Soften the tortilla in a microwave for 15 seconds or in a nonstick skillet for about 30 seconds on each side. Spread the refried beans over the tortilla and place on a plate.

Beat the egg with the salt, Tabasco, and 1 teaspoon of cold water. Heat the oil in a nonstick skillet over medium-high heat. Pour in the egg mixture and stir briefly until it begins to thicken, about 1 minute. Turn off the heat and continue to scramble the egg, folding large curds over, until just set, about 1 minute longer. Spoon onto the tortilla.

Top with the cheese, salsa, and scallion. Roll up and eat slowly, chewing well to savor every tasty bite.

Cherry-Apple Oatmeal

Good fiber and powerful antioxidants are combined in this yummy breakfast cereal. Serve with ½ cup soy milk or whole or 2 percent cow's milk. Both rice and almond milk have significantly less protein, but you can use them if you prefer. Add half a grapefruit or a small orange for a complete breakfast. Because this recipe makes two servings, you can split it with another person, or save the extra half and reheat it in the microwave the next day.

½ cup steel-cut oats	1 small tart apple, cored and finely diced (peeling is optional)	1½ tablespoons dried cherries, coarsely chopped if large
2 cups water		
Pinch of salt		

Put the oats in a 1½-quart saucepan with the 2 cups water and a pinch of salt. Slowly bring to a boil.

Add the apple and dried cherries to the oatmeal and decrease the heat to a bare simmer. Partially cover the pot and cook until most of the water is absorbed and the oats are tender but still have a pleasing texture, 12 to 15 minutes.

Note: You can make this same oatmeal with regular rolled oats. If you do so, cooking time will be about 5 minutes less.

Mexican Scrambled Eggs

Traditionally, this is made with stale corn tortillas. Ready-made tortilla chips are even easier. For brunch, offer an assortment of condiments on the side: guacamole, sour cream, and shredded cheese.

4 eggs	2 tablespoons extra-virgin olive oil	1½ tablespoons chopped pickled jalapeños
2 or 3 dashes of Tabasco sauce	½ teaspoon ground cumin	2 ounces corn tortilla chips, coarsely broken
Salt and freshly ground pepper	¾ cup chopped tomato	
½ onion, finely chopped		

In a bowl, beat the eggs lightly. Season with the Tabasco and salt and pepper to taste.

continued

In a nonstick skillet, cook the onion in the olive oil over medium-high heat until softened and beginning to color around the edges, about 5 minutes.

Sprinkle on the cumin and cook for another 30 seconds. Add the tomato and jalapeños and cook, stirring occasionally, until the tomatoes soften, about 3 minutes. Decrease the heat to low.

Pour in the eggs and scramble, folding from the bottom of the pan with a silicone or wooden spatula, until the eggs are almost set. Add the tortilla chips, remove from the heat, and stir to mix and finish setting the eggs. Let stand for 2 minutes, then serve.

Eggs Florentine

4 SERVINGS | 9 POINTS EACH

Using an egg-poaching mold makes preparation much easier. If you use a mold, you can omit the vinegar.

1 Polenta Crouton (page 213) or ½ lightly toasted high-fiber whole grain English muffin	2 teaspoons distilled white vinegar	1½ cups (lightly packed) baby spinach
	1 very fresh egg	Salt and freshly ground pepper
1 slice (½ to 1 ounce) Swiss, Gruyère, Cheddar, or Manchego cheese	1 teaspoon minced shallot	1 thin slice smoked salmon (½ ounce; optional)
	1 tablespoon extra-virgin olive oil	

Preheat the broiler. Put the polenta crouton on a sheet of aluminum foil, top with the cheese, and broil for 1 to 2 minutes, until the cheese is melted.

Bring a small saucepan of salted water to a boil over medium-high heat, then add the vinegar. Decrease the heat to a bare simmer. Crack the egg into a saucer and gently slide it into the water. Cook for 1 minute, folding any white that slips away up and over the egg. Cover the pot and cook until the white is firm and the yolk still runny, about 3 more minutes. Use a slotted spoon or skimmer to remove the poached egg and set it on a plate.

Meanwhile, in a nonstick skillet over medium heat, cook the shallot in the olive oil until soft, about 2 minutes. Raise the heat to medium-high, toss in the spinach, and cook, tossing, until just wilted, 10 to 15 seconds. Immediately remove from the heat and season lightly with salt and pepper.

To assemble the dish, put the cheese crouton on a plate. Arrange the sautéed spinach on the crouton, letting it spill over onto the plate. Add the smoked salmon. Top with the poached egg and serve at once.

Smoked Turkey Hash

4 SERVINGS | 14 POINTS EACH

Turkey hash is a natural during the holidays when you have a big leftover bird in the fridge, so feel free to make this same recipe with plain turkey, if you wish. But any day of the year, you can buy the smoked variety in the deli section. The vegetables can be steamed the night before. If you happen to have leftover cooked vegetables, by all means use those. Serve the hash as is, or with a poached egg on top. We also like a dollop of ketchup on the side.

10 ounces smoked turkey, sliced ½ inch thick

2 Yukon gold potatoes, cut into ½-inch dice

1 large carrot, peeled and cut into ½-inch dice

10 brussels sprouts, halved or quartered

1 onion, coarsely chopped

2 tablespoons extra-virgin olive oil

½ teaspoon dried thyme

Sea salt and freshly ground pepper

½ cup chicken stock or reduced-sodium canned broth

2 teaspoons Worcestershire sauce

½ teaspoon Tabasco sauce or other hot sauce

Cut the turkey into ½-inch dice; set aside.

Put the potatoes, carrot, and brussels sprouts on a steamer rack. Set over boiling water and steam until the vegetables are just tender, 3 to 4 minutes. Remove immediately. Rinse under cold running water to stop the cooking; drain well.

In a large skillet, cook the onion in the olive oil over medium heat, covered, for 3 minutes to soften. Uncover, increase the heat to medium-high, and sauté, stirring occasionally until golden, 3 to 4 minutes.

Add the turkey and vegetables. Season with the thyme, 1 teaspoon of salt, and ¼ teaspoon of pepper. Toss over the heat for 2 to 3 minutes. Add the chicken stock, Worcestershire, and hot sauce. Continue to cook, tossing, until the hash is almost dry. Season with additional salt and pepper to taste.

Crunchy Cranberry Granola

MAKES 1½ CUPS; 6 SERVINGS | 6 POINTS EACH

Most commercially produced granola is laden with fat and sugar. This one provides the same toasty crunch along with plenty of fiber and only a hint of natural sweetness. A few tablespoons of this granola makes a satisfying snack, and a light sprinkling transforms plain yogurt or fresh fruit into something special.

1 tablespoon freshly squeezed orange juice

1 tablespoon brown rice syrup or honey

1 tablespoon sunflower oil

½ teaspoon vanilla extract

¼ teaspoon ground cinnamon

⅛ teaspoon salt

1 cup rolled oats

2 tablespoons sliced almonds

2 tablespoons roasted, unsalted sunflower seeds

1 tablespoon unsweetened coconut flakes

2 tablespoons dried cranberries

Preheat the oven to 300°F. Coat a baking sheet with nonstick cooking spray.

In a bowl, combine the orange juice, brown rice syrup, oil, vanilla, cinnamon, and salt. Mix until well blended. Add the oats, almonds, sunflower seeds, and coconut flakes and stir until evenly moistened. Spread the mixture in a thin, even layer on the prepared baking sheet.

Bake, stirring once or twice, until fragrant and golden, 15 to 20 minutes. Stir in the dried cranberries and let cool completely. Use at once, or store in an airtight container for up to 1 week.

Whole Grain Griddle Cakes

6 SERVINGS | 16 POINTS EACH

This recipe is offered as a treat, not an everyday meal. Allow 3 cakes per person. Since that alone won't feel like nearly enough, accompany with a fruit salad and maybe a small serving of yogurt. Or really splurge and have a couple of slices of lean, nitrate-free bacon.

1 cup white whole wheat or whole wheat flour

½ cup fine cornmeal

⅓ cup buckwheat flour

4 teaspoon turbinado or demerara sugar

1 teaspoon baking powder

¾ teaspoon baking soda

½ teaspoon salt

2 eggs

2 cups buttermilk

2 tablespoons unsalted butter, melted and slightly cooled

2 tablespoons canola or soybean oil

In a bowl, combine the white wheat flour, cornmeal, buckwheat flour, sugar, baking powder, baking soda, and salt. Whisk gently to blend. Set the dry ingredients aside.

In another bowl, whisk the eggs to break them up. Gradually beat in the buttermilk and mix well. Beat in the melted butter.

Add the liquids to the dry ingredients and stir just until blended; do not overmix.

To cook the griddle cakes, heat about 1 tablespoon of the oil in a large heavy skillet or griddle. Ladle 3 to 4 tablespoons of batter into the pan per cake. Cook until most of the bubbles that form on top break and the bottom is golden brown, about 3 minutes. Flip over and cook until spotted brown on the other side, about 1 minute. Remove to a platter. Adjust the heat as necessary so that the griddle cakes cook through without burning. Repeat with the remaining oil and batter.

Egyptian Breakfast Beans

4 SERVINGS | 5 POINTS EACH

Many of us have rather set ideas of what constitutes a morning meal, but in other parts of the world people eat a variety of breakfast foods. One of the healthiest, especially for modulating blood sugar, is the Middle Eastern *ful medames*, **stewed fava beans, often served with yogurt or feta cheese, chopped vegetables, and a hard-boiled egg. If you have the points, a whole wheat pita would round out the meal.**

3 tablespoons extra-virgin olive oil	1 cup chopped fresh plum tomatoes (1½ large or 3 small)	1 tablespoon freshly squeezed lemon juice
½ onion, finely chopped	4 teaspoons Aleppo pepper or ⅛ teaspoon crushed hot red pepper	1 teaspoon coarse (kosher) salt
3 cloves garlic: 2 minced, 1 crushed through a press	1 (15-ounce) can fava beans, drained and rinsed	3 hard-boiled eggs, peeled and halved or quartered lengthwise
1 teaspoon ground cumin		2 tablespoons finely chopped parsley

In a large saucepan, heat 2 tablespoons of the olive oil over medium heat. Add the onion and cook until soft and beginning to turn golden, about 5 minutes. Add the 2 minced garlic cloves and the cumin and cook for 30 seconds. Add the tomatoes and Aleppo pepper and continue to cook, stirring occasionally, until they soften and give up their liquid, 3 to 5 minutes.

Add the beans and 1 cup of water. Bring to a boil. Decrease the heat and simmer, stirring and mashing some of the beans with a fork, until they are coarsely crushed, about 5 minutes.

continued

Use an old-fashioned potato masher or a fork to mash the beans into a coarse puree. Add a little more water if you need to. Remove from the heat. Stir in the lemon juice, the crushed garlic clove, and the remaining 1 tablespoon of olive oil. Season with additional salt to taste. Arrange the *ful* on a platter or plates and garnish with the eggs and parsley.

Note: To boil an egg perfectly, put it in a small saucepan and add water to cover. Bring just to a boil, turn off the heat, and cover. Let stand exactly 15 minutes for hard-cooked eggs, 13 to 14 minutes for medium eggs (with the yolk not fully set), and 12 minutes for soft-boiled eggs.

Italian Vegetable Frittata

6 SERVINGS | 8 POINTS EACH

A frittata is much like an omelet, but it's thicker and denser. You can add almost anything you like to the eggs, but potatoes and onions usually form the base. You can enjoy it warm, at room temperature, or chilled, which makes it a great choice for a picnic.

3 tablespoons extra-virgin olive oil	1 onion, cut into ½-inch dice	¾ cup lightly steamed broccoli florets
2 small Yukon gold potatoes, peeled and cut into ¼-inch slices	¾ cup diced (½-inch) red bell pepper	3 tablespoons cream cheese (1½ ounces)
Salt and freshly ground pepper	7 eggs	2 to 3 tablespoons shredded Parmesan or Manchego cheese
	2 or 3 dashes of Tabasco sauce	

In a well-seasoned 9-inch cast-iron or ovenproof nonstick skillet, heat 1½ table-spoons of the olive oil. Add the potatoes, cover, and cook over medium heat, turning them once or twice, until tender and golden brown, 6 to 8 minutes. Season generously with salt and pepper. Transfer the potatoes to a plate.

Heat the remaining 1½ tablespoons of oil in the skillet, swirling to coat the sides of the pan. Add the onion and cook over medium-high heat until it is softened and just beginning to brown, 3 to 5 minutes. Add the diced pepper, decrease the heat to medium, and cook until softened, about 3 minutes longer. Return the potatoes to the pan.

Beat the eggs until blended. Season with the Tabasco and a generous pinch of salt and pepper. Pour into the skillet, tilting the pan so the egg covers the vegetables evenly. Decrease the heat to medium-low. Lift the edges of the frittata and let the uncooked egg flow underneath. Arrange the broccoli florets on top.

Dollop bits of the cream cheese in between the vegetables. Cover and cook until the frittata is set around the edges but still runny in the center, 3 to 5 minutes.

Sprinkle the Parmesan cheese over the top. Transfer to the broiler and cook 4 to 6 inches from the heat until the frittata is puffed and very lightly browned on top, 2 to 3 minutes.

Asparagus Frittata with Goat Cheese

4 SERVINGS | 6 POINTS EACH

When tender young asparagus appears at the market, it's a sign that spring has officially begun. Celebrate the season with a frittata that's simple enough for a quick family meal, yet elegant enough for company.

6 eggs

½ teaspoon salt

¼ teaspoon freshly ground pepper

2 tablespoons extra-virgin olive oil

1 shallot, finely chopped

8 ounces asparagus, trimmed and cut into 2-inch pieces

½ cup crumbled soft goat cheese (about 2 ounces)

2 tablespoons coarsely torn or chopped fresh mint leaves or parsley

Preheat the oven broiler.

In a bowl, combine the eggs, salt, and pepper. Whisk until blended.

Heat the oil in a 10-inch skillet (preferably nonstick with an ovenproof handle), turning to coat the bottom and sides with oil. Add the shallot and cook over medium heat, stirring, until softened but not browned, about 3 minutes. Add the asparagus and increase the heat to medium-high. Cook, stirring and tossing, until the asparagus turns bright green, 1 to 2 minutes.

Decrease the heat to medium and spread the asparagus and shallot in an even layer. Carefully pour in the eggs and cook, using a spatula to lift the edges as they firm up to let the uncooked egg flow under, until the underside is fully set but the center is still slightly runny. Shake the pan now and then to make sure the frittata is loose and not sticking.

Scatter the cheese over the top. Place the frittata under the broiler, watching carefully, until the cheese has softened and the top is very lightly browned, 1 to 2 minutes. Slide the frittata onto a warm serving plate and sprinkle the mint over the top. Serve warm, cut into wedges.

SMOOTHIES

Smoothies are incredibly popular these days, and I can't help suspecting the hip pizzazz of the name has something to do with it. A creamy iced beverage somehow links health and simplicity of preparation with a bikini-ready body and maybe a surfboard on the side.

It's true, a properly designed drink can provide an easy source of protein and calcium in the A.M., as well as at least two of your vegetable and fruit servings. But it's important to keep in mind that it can also be a huge calorie sink. Protein powders offer unnecessarily large doses of protein along with extra calories you don't need. Likewise, although bananas are a good source of potassium, they are also relatively high in carbohydrates and sugar, so they should be included judiciously. I recommend you get your complete protein from soy or cow's milk and yogurt.

Keep in mind, too, that this healthy beverage will not give you the same feeling of satisfaction as solid food. Your body reacts differently to liquids, even thick ones. So you'll want some other food to keep you going: one egg, a small bowl of oatmeal, or a small slice of whole grain bread with cheese.

Most of these recipes make a generous 2 cups. This can be enough to share with someone else, or you can drink half for breakfast and take along the other half for a nice snack when you start to flag in the middle of the morning.

Strawberry Magic Smoothie

2 SERVINGS | 10 POINTS EACH

Smoothies are a great way to slip in an extra vegetable serving. Here the vitamin C in the strawberries will help you absorb the minerals in the kale. Use frozen berries or serve over ice if you like your smoothie extra chilled.

⅔ cup plain soy milk

½ cup cold water

3 ounces (about ⅓ cup) plain whole-milk yogurt, preferably goat's milk yogurt, or reduced-fat Greek yogurt

¾ cup cut-up fresh or frozen strawberries

½ cup packed shredded lacinato or red kale leaves (stems removed) or baby kale

1 tablespoon sliced almonds

2 teaspoons peeled, thinly sliced fresh ginger

½ teaspoon vanilla extract

2 to 3 teaspoons maple syrup

Combine all the ingredients in a blender or food processor. Puree for 1 to 2 minutes, until completely smooth and creamy, stopping to scrape down the sides as needed.

A Berry Berry Morning

2 SERVINGS | 6 POINTS EACH

If your berries are ripe and sweet, you won't need any sugar here. But since fruit is so inconsistent, especially out of season, if the berries are tart, you have the option of adding 1 to 2 teaspoons of sugar, maple syrup, or honey.

6 ounces (about ⅔ cup) plain whole-milk yogurt, preferably goat's milk yogurt

½ cup soy milk

½ cup fresh or frozen raspberries

½ cup cut-up fresh or frozen strawberries

½ cup crushed ice (if using fresh berries) or ⅓ cup cold water (if using frozen)

1 tablespoon sliced almonds

¼ teaspoon almond extract

¼ teaspoon vanilla extract

1 to 2 teaspoons sugar, maple syrup, or honey (optional)

Combine the yogurt, milk, raspberries, strawberries, ice, almonds, and extracts in a blender or food processor. Puree for 1 to 2 minutes, until completely smooth and creamy, stopping to scrape down the sides as needed. Add the sugar, ½ teaspoon at a time, to taste.

Blueberry Lemon Frost

2 GENEROUS SERVINGS | 5 POINTS EACH

This is a light, pleasing smoothie that needs no added sweetener if the fruit is ripe enough. Because rice milk contains almost no protein, one serving of this with the yogurt will contribute only 3 or 4 grams of protein, which makes it a better choice for a snack rather than a meal substitute. If you want it for breakfast, have a boiled or poached egg on the side. Or use soy milk rather than rice milk to triple the protein.

1 cup rice milk

6 ounces (about ⅔ cup) plain goat's milk yogurt or full-fat or reduced-fat Greek yogurt

1 cup packed fresh torn spinach leaves or baby spinach

¾ cup fresh or frozen blueberries

1 small or ¾ medium ripe banana (⅓ cup mashed)

Zest and juice of ½ lemon

½ teaspoon ground cinnamon

⅛ teaspoon freshly grated nutmeg

½ cup crushed ice (if using fresh berries) or ⅓ cold water (if using frozen)

Combine all the ingredients in a blender or food processor. Puree for 1 to 2 minutes, until completely smooth and creamy, stopping to scrape down the sides as needed.

Peach-Almond Smoothie

1 SERVING | 8 POINTS

When your refrigerator is overflowing with all the summer fruit you couldn't resist at the farmers' market, this is a delicious way to use up any that may be turning soft. During the rest of the year, frozen fruit is the way to go.

1 cup chopped peaches, fresh or frozen and partially thawed

2 ounces (about ¼ cup) plain whole-milk yogurt, preferably goat's milk yogurt

½ cup cold water

1 tablespoon sliced almonds

2 teaspoons brown rice syrup or honey

¼ teaspoon almond extract

Combine all the ingredients in a blender or food processor. Puree for 1 to 2 minutes, until completely smooth and creamy, stopping to scrape down the sides as needed. Serve over ice.

Tropical Mango Smoothie

1 SERVING | 7 POINTS

A touch of uncooked oatmeal, though imperceptible, adds a bit more fiber to this luxurious blend. Be sure to shake the can of coconut milk before opening, so the rich cream that rises to the top in storage is distributed throughout.

1 cup peeled and diced mango, fresh or frozen and partially thawed

¾ cup soy milk

1 tablespoon quick-cooking or old-fashioned rolled oats (oatmeal)

1 tablespoon freshly squeezed lime juice

1 teaspoon brown sugar

Combine all the ingredients in a blender or food processor. Puree for 1 to 2 minutes, until completely smooth and creamy, stopping to scrape down the sides as needed. Serve over ice.

SOUPS AND CHOWDERS

Soup offers a great way to assemble a light meal or to fill up a bit before your main course. As you'll see, homemade soup is easy and not nearly as time-consuming as you might think.

Cod-Corn Chowder

6 SERVINGS | 16 POINTS EACH

Accompany this meal-in-a-bowl with a side of coleslaw or a kale salad.

2 ounces diced pancetta (about ¼ cup)

2 tablespoons unsalted butter

2 tablespoons extra-virgin olive oil

1 onion, chopped

½ fresh fennel bulb, diced

3 tablespoons all-purpose flour

2 cups fish stock, or 1 cup clam juice mixed with 1 cup water

1½ cups peeled and diced (½ inch) Yukon gold potatoes (about 2)

1 medium-large leek (white and tender green parts), diced and well rinsed

1 teaspoon thyme

Dash each of Worcestershire sauce and Tabasco sauce

1½ cups whole milk

12 ounces skinless cod fillet or "tenderloins," cut into 1-inch chunks

⅓ cup heavy cream or half-and-half

Kernels from 2 ears of corn or 1 cup canned or frozen corn

Salt and freshly ground pepper

In a large pot, cook the pancetta in the butter and oil over medium heat until it renders most of its fat, 3 to 4 minutes. Transfer to a small bowl with a slotted spoon.

Add the onion to the fat in the pot and cook over medium heat until softened and just beginning to turn golden, 5 to 7 minutes. Add the fennel and cook for 3 minutes more.

Sprinkle on the flour and cook, stirring, for about 2 minutes without allowing the flour to color. Whisk in the stock and bring to a boil, continuing to whisk until evenly mixed.

Add the potatoes, leek, thyme, Worcestershire, and Tabasco. Pour in the milk. Bring to a boil again and cook until the potatoes are just tender, about 5 minutes.

Add the cod, cream, and corn, decrease the heat to a simmer, and cook for 5 minutes longer, breaking up the cod into large flakes. Season with salt and pepper to taste. Serve hot.

Cardamom-Scented Butternut Squash Soup with Lemon Cream

6 SERVINGS | 7 POINTS EACH

This recipe is a simplified version of a sumptuous soup served at L'Astrance, a three-star restaurant in Paris. You can make it with all water, but the chicken broth adds an extra depth of flavor.

1 butternut squash (1½ to 1¾ pounds)

2 tablespoons extra-virgin olive oil

1 leek (white and tender green parts), thinly sliced

1½ teaspoons freshly crushed green cardamom, or 1 teaspoon ground cardamom and 1 teaspoon ground coriander

1 teaspoon turbinado or brown sugar

⅛ teaspoon cayenne pepper

2½ cups chicken broth diluted with 2½ cups water

Zest and juice of ½ lemon

Salt and freshly ground pepper

Lemon Cream (recipe follows)

Preheat the oven to 400°F. Prick the squash in a few places, set in a shallow baking dish, and roast until soft and browned outside, about 45 minutes. When the squash is cool enough to handle, cut it in half and scoop out the seeds. Peel off the outer skin.

Warm the olive oil in a large saucepan over medium heat. Add the leek and cook, stirring once or twice, until soft but not brown, 3 to 5 minutes. Add the cardamom and cook for 1 minute.

Add the roasted squash to the pot and stir, mashing it up a bit. Add the sugar and cayenne. Pour in the broth and water. Bring to a boil, decrease the heat to medium-low, partially cover, and simmer for 15 minutes.

Puree the soup with an immersion blender or transfer to a food processer or blender and puree until smooth. Stir in the lemon zest and juice. Season with salt and pepper to taste. Serve hot, with a dollop of lemon cream on top.

Lemon Cream

MAKES ABOUT ½ CUP; 6 SERVINGS | 1½ POINTS EACH

With its hit of lemon zest, this cream really brightens up the butternut soup.

Zest of ½ lemon

¼ cup full-fat sour cream

2 ounces (about ¼ cup) plain whole-milk yogurt, preferably goat's milk yogurt

In a small bowl, stir together the lemon zest, sour cream, and yogurt until well blended.

Cheddared Broccoli Soup

6 SERVINGS | 8 POINTS EACH

Broccoli soup takes on a subtle but substantial dimension with the addition of cheese. Choose the best-quality, sharpest Cheddar you can find and be sure to stir it in after the soup is off the heat so it doesn't toughen.

---

1 large bunch broccoli, 1½ to 2 pounds

3 tablespoons extra-virgin olive oil

2 onions, sliced

2 tablespoons all-purpose flour

6 cups chicken broth

¼ cup heavy cream

1 tablespoon freshly squeezed lemon juice

1 teaspoon Worcestershire sauce

Salt

Tabasco sauce

4 ounces extra-sharp Cheddar cheese, shredded (about 1 cup)

Trim the ends off the broccoli. Peel the thick stems and cut into 1-inch chunks; set aside. Separate the crowns into 1-inch florets; keep separate from the stems.

In a large flameproof casserole or heavy soup pot, heat the olive oil and cook the onions, covered, over low heat for 5 minutes. Uncover, increase the heat to medium, and cook, stirring occasionally, until they are soft and just beginning to color, another 5 to 7 minutes.

Sprinkle in the flour and cook, stirring, for 1 to 2 minutes. Gradually whisk in the broth. Bring to a boil. Add the broccoli stems and cook over medium-high heat for 3 minutes. Add the broccoli florets and cook until tender but still bright green, about 3 to 4 minutes longer.

Puree the soup in the pot with an immersion blender, or transfer to a blender or food processor in batches, puree until smooth, and return to the pot.

Stir in the cream, lemon juice, and Worcestershire sauce. Simmer uncovered for 5 minutes. Season with salt and Tabasco to taste. Remove from the heat and stir in the cheese until melted. Serve hot.

Chilled Avocado and Cucumber Soup

4 SERVINGS | 3 POINTS EACH

Avocados are nutrient-rich, offering a good source of healthy monounsaturated fats, vitamin E, folate, and potassium, among other good things. Quick, easy, and satisfying, this soup is delicious enough for company.

1 large (English) seedless cucumber or 2 large regular cucumbers 2 ripe avocados	1½ cups plain chicken stock, soy milk, or rice milk 2 tablespoons freshly squeezed lemon juice	3 tablespoons chopped fresh dill Sea salt and freshly ground pepper

Peel the cucumber(s); scoop out and discard any seeds. Cut the cucumbers into chunks and put in a food processor or blender.

Halve the avocados and remove the pits. Using a large spoon, scoop the avocado flesh into the food processor and discard the skin.

Add the stock, lemon juice, and 2 tablespoons of the dill. Puree until smooth. Season with salt and pepper to taste. Transfer to a covered container and refrigerate just until chilled. Check the seasonings again before serving, and add more salt and pepper to tast. Garnish with the remaining 1 tablespoon of dill.

Lemony Escarole and Rice Soup

4 SERVINGS | 3 POINTS EACH

Light soups provide an excellent way to fill up with low-calorie liquids and get plenty of vegetables. Serve with a small extra drizzle of olive oil, if you like, and a tablespoon of grated cheese.

3 cloves garlic, chopped 2 tablespoons extra-virgin olive oil Pinch of crushed hot red pepper	1 large head escarole, torn up and well rinsed 6 cups chicken or vegetable stock	1 cup cooked imported brown basmati rice 2 tablespoons freshly squeezed lemon juice Salt and freshly ground pepper

In a soup pot, cook the garlic in the olive oil over medium heat until it just starts to color. Add the hot red pepper and escarole and stir to coat with the oil.

Pour in the stock, bring to a boil, and cook until the escarole is tender, about 10 minutes. Stir in the rice and lemon juice. Season with salt and pepper to taste and serve.

Cream of Tomato Soup with Basil and Mint

6 SERVINGS | 10 POINTS EACH

Fresh basil and mint add piquancy and an herbaceous accent to this easy, creamy tomato soup. Use canned tomatoes or preferably Pomi brand, which comes in a Tetra Pak box and contains no additives.

1 large leek (white and pale green parts), sliced and well rinsed

2 cloves garlic, minced

3 tablespoons extra-virgin olive oil

2 tablespoons all-purpose flour

2 cups chicken broth

1 (28-ounce) can chopped tomatoes with their juices

⅓ cup fresh basil leaves

¼ cup fresh mint leaves

½ cup heavy cream

Salt and cayenne pepper

In a large saucepan or soup pot, cook the leek and garlic in the olive oil over medium heat until softened but not browned, 3 to 5 minutes. Sprinkle on the flour and cook, stirring, for 1 to 2 minutes without letting the flour color. Pour in the broth and bring to a boil, whisking as it thickens so there are no lumps. Decrease the heat and simmer for 5 minutes.

Meanwhile, puree the tomatoes with the basil and mint until smooth. Stir into the soup base. Return to a simmer and continue to cook for 10 minutes longer.

Stir in the cream and heat through. Season with salt and cayenne pepper to taste.

Mushroom-Barley Soup

6 SERVINGS | 4 POINTS EACH

Barley has the same healthy type of fiber as oatmeal; it slows carbohydrate absorption and helps reduce cholesterol. A cup of soup as a first course can take the edge off your hunger, so portion control is easier when you get to the main event. A bowlful can make a satisfying lunch, with a salad on the side. If you have access to assorted varieties of fresh mushrooms, by all means use a mixture for added depth of flavor. This recipe freezes well, so homemade soup can always be just minutes away.

½ cup pearl barley

2 tablespoons extra-virgin olive oil

2 onions, chopped

3 celery ribs, chopped

1 carrot, thinly sliced

1½ pounds mushrooms, sliced

4 cups beef, chicken, or vegetable broth

2 cups (packed) baby spinach leaves, cut into ¼-inch strips or chopped

1 teaspoon soy sauce

Salt and freshly ground pepper

continued

In a large saucepan, combine the barley with 4 cups of water. Bring to a boil over medium-high heat and cook, partially covered, until the barley is just softened but only about half cooked, 15 to 20 minutes.

Meanwhile, in a large flameproof casserole, heat the oil over medium heat. Add the onions, celery, and carrot and cook, stirring occasionally, until softened, 7 to 9 minutes. Stir in the mushrooms and cook until they begin to release their liquid, about 5 minutes.

Pour in the barley and its cooking liquid and add the broth. Bring to a boil, then decrease the heat to medium-low and cook, partially covered and stirring occasionally, until the barley is tender, about 20 minutes.

Stir in the spinach and soy sauce. Season with salt and pepper to taste. Serve at once, or let cool to room temperature and refrigerate or freeze.

Turnip and Mustard Green Soup with Pinto Beans and Ham

6 SERVINGS | 7 POINTS EACH

This is a fabulous savory winter soup. Processed meats are not favored on our budget, but ½ ounce per serving is fine for a special treat.

1 large sweet onion, diced

3 tablespoons extra-virgin olive oil

2 turnips, peeled and diced

2 large carrots, peeled and diced

4 ounces lean nitrate-free ham, cut ½ inch thick and diced

10 cups water

2 large cubes or 2 tablespoons vegetable bouillon, preferably imported, such as Rapunzel brand

1 dried chipotle chile

1 bunch mustard greens, stemmed and torn into pieces (6 to 8 cups)

1 (15-ounce) can pinto beans, rinsed and drained

Salt and freshly ground pepper

In a soup pot over medium heat, cook the onion in the olive oil for 3 minutes to soften. Uncover, raise the heat to medium-high, and cook until golden around the edges, about 3 minutes longer.

Add the turnips, carrots, and ham to the pot and sauté, stirring, for 2 to 3 minutes. Pour in the water, add the vegetable bouillon and the dried chile, and bring to a boil. Decrease the heat and simmer for 5 minutes.

Add the mustard greens and return to a simmer. Cook, partially covered, until the greens are just tender, about 10 minutes. Add the beans and heat through. Season with salt and pepper to taste. Discard the chile before serving.

Italian Minestrone

6 SERVINGS | 9 POINTS EACH

Here's the classic recipe at its most basic. If you like, feel free to add diced cabbage, celery, and fresh fennel along with the other vegetables.

1 onion, chopped

3 tablespoons extra-virgin olive oil

2 tablespoons tomato paste

1 (14.5-ounce) can diced tomatoes with their juices

¾ cup diced peeled carrots

¾ cup diced peeled Yukon gold potatoes

¾ cup diced green beans

¼ cup chopped fresh basil, or 1½ teaspoons dried oregano

2 cups chicken broth

3 cups (lightly packed) shredded kale or chard

1 (15-ounce) can cannellini beans, rinsed and drained

Salt and freshly ground pepper

More extra-virgin olive oil and grated Romano or Parmesan cheese, for sprinkling

In a large soup pot, cook the onion in the olive oil over medium heat, covered, for 3 minutes, to soften. Uncover, raise the heat to medium-high, and continue to cook until the onion is just beginning to color, about 3 minutes longer.

Add the tomato paste and cook, stirring, until the paste darkens slightly, 1 to 2 minutes. Pour in the diced tomatoes and stir to mix. Add the carrots, potatoes, green beans, and basil. Pour in the broth and add 4 cups of water. Bring to a boil and cook over medium-high heat for 15 minutes.

Add the kale and cannellini beans and cook for 5 to 10 minutes longer, until the kale is just tender. Season with salt and pepper to taste.

Ladle into soup bowls and pass a cruet of olive oil and a bowl of grated cheese at the table.

FISH AND OTHER SEAFOOD

One of the healthiest changes you can make is to increase your fish consumption to twice a week. Remember, canned tuna, salmon, and sardines count. A serving of bone-in sardines has almost as much calcium as a glass of milk. And salmon is a good source of B$_{12}$ and iron for people avoiding red meat.

Flounder with Almonds and Lemon Butter

2 SERVINGS | 22 POINTS EACH

This dish is traditionally made with fillet of sole, a flat fish like flounder, but sole is hard to come by these days. Flounder, especially locally caught, makes a fine substitute. For a crisp coating, dredge the fish in the flour just before you add it to the pan.

2 flounder or sole fillets (about 4 ounces each)	2 tablespoons extra-virgin olive oil	2 teaspoons finely minced shallots
⅓ cup all-purpose flour	3 tablespoons unsalted butter	1 tablespoon freshly squeezed lemon juice
¼ teaspoon salt	3 tablespoons sliced almonds	Lemon wedges, for garnish
⅛ teaspoon freshly ground pepper		

Pat the fish dry. Place the flour on a plate or in a shallow bowl and season with salt and pepper. Dredge the fish in the flour to coat both sides.

Heat the oil and 1 tablespoon of the butter in a large heavy skillet over medium-high heat until the butter melts and the foam subsides. Add the fish fillets and sauté, turning once with a wide spatula, until browned and just cooked through, about 2 minutes per side. Remove to a plate.

Pour the fat out of the pan and carefully wipe with a folded paper towel. Add the remaining 2 tablespoons butter and set the pan on medium heat. Add the almonds and shallots and cook, stirring, until the almonds are just golden brown and the shallots are softened, about 2 minutes.

Immediately remove from the heat and pour in the lemon juice. Pour the sauce and toasted almonds over the fish, garnish with the lemon wedges, and serve at once.

Salmon-Stuffed Cabbage with Savory Lentils

4 SERVINGS | 18 POINTS EACH

This exquisite dish is not difficult, but it does have a few steps, so it might best be reserved for weekends. It's satisfying enough for Sunday supper and elegant enough for a dinner party. To make it easy on yourself, prepare the lentils and parboil the cabbage leaves up to a day in advance. You can also assemble the dish entirely several hours ahead, refrigerate, and then bake it shortly before serving.

---

12 ounces center-cut salmon fillet, skinned

1 teaspoon ground coriander

½ teaspoon salt

⅛ teaspoon freshly ground pepper

1 lemon, cut into quarters

Savory Lentils with Mushrooms and Dill (page 205)

1 large head savoy cabbage

1½ teaspoons tomato paste

¾ cup hot chicken or vegetable stock

1 teaspoon turbinado or light brown sugar

Season the salmon with the ground coriander, salt, pepper, and the juice from 1 quarter of the lemon. Divide the salmon into 4 equal pieces. Refrigerate until ready to use.

If you haven't prepared them in advance, make one batch of the savory lentils. Preheat the oven to 375°F.

Bring a large pot of salted water to a boil. Remove and discard any dark green leaves on the outside of the cabbage. Peel off 10 to 12 of the largest remaining leaves. Add the whole cabbage leaves to the boiling water and cook until they are just tender and pliable but not mushy, 6 or 7 minutes. Remove and immediately rinse under cold running water. Finely slice the remaining cabbage.

Cut off the tough stems from the cooked cabbage leaves, leaving them as intact as possible. Overlap 2 of the cabbage leaves, veined side down. Place one piece of salmon in the center. Top with ¼ cup of the savory lentils. Wrap up in the inner leaf; then fold up in the outer leaf so the filling is completely enclosed. Repeat with the remaining cabbage, salmon, and lentils.

In a shallow baking dish large enough to hold all the cabbage rolls, make a bed of the sliced cabbage. In a small bowl, stir the tomato paste into the juice of the remaining 3 lemon quarters. Mix in the stock and the sugar. Pour over the cabbage. Arrange the cabbage rolls in the dish.

Cover with foil and bake for 25 minutes. Uncover and bake for 15 to 20 minutes more, until the salmon is just cooked through and opaque in the center. Serve each cabbage roll with some of the shredded cabbage and sauce.

Chinese-Style Steamed Black Bass with Ginger, Leeks, and Mushrooms

4 SERVINGS | 16 POINTS EACH

This dish is best made with a fine-textured white fish like sea bass; other good choices are striped bass or red snapper. You can also use salmon, but if you do so, allow an extra 3 to 5 minutes cooking time. If your fish is really fresh, there is no better way to cook it than steaming, which poaches the delicate meat while retaining all the moisture and flavor. The warm sauce is poured over the fish just before serving. Serve with steamed broccoli rabe or baby broccoli and a small portion of brown rice.

---

12 to 16 ounces black sea bass fillet

1 tablespoon (packed) finely shredded fresh ginger

1 small leek (white and tender green parts), thinly sliced lengthwise, or 2 scallions, cut into 2-inch lengths

4 to 6 white button mushrooms, sliced paper-thin

2 cups fresh tender pea shoots or baby spinach

1½ tablespoons peanut oil or extra-virgin olive oil

1½ tablespoons toasted sesame oil

2 tablespoons soy sauce or wheat-free tamari

Run your fingers over the meaty side of the fish to check for any bones. If you find any, use a sturdy tweezers to pull them out cleanly.

Arrange the fish on a steamer rack, skin side down. Spread the ginger over the fillet, then sprinkle the leek evenly over the fish. Top with slices of mushroom to cover.

Bring about an inch of water to a boil in the bottom of the steamer. Set the rack in place, cover, and steam for 5 minutes. Plop the pea shoots over the fillet, cover, and steam for 2 minutes longer. Transfer the fish to a deep platter.

While the fish is steaming, in a small saucepan, combine the peanut oil, sesame oil, and soy sauce. Warm until hot. Pour the hot sauce over the fish and serve.

Salmon Cupcakes with Cucumber-Yogurt Sauce

No one can deny the convenience of nutrient-rich canned salmon, and now canned wild salmon, with better flavor and more omega-3s, is readily available in supermarkets. Here salmon cakes are given a deliciously whimsical treatment, baked in the shape of cupcakes and topped with a dollop of tangy cucumber-yogurt sauce. *Note:* The sauce must be started at least a day in advance.

---

1 large can (14.75 ounces) wild Alaska salmon

1 slice 100 percent whole wheat bread, torn into pieces (about 1 ounce)

2 tablespoons quick-cooking or old-fashioned rolled oats

2 eggs

¼ teaspoon salt

2½ tablespoons mayonnaise

1 teaspoon Dijon mustard

¼ teaspoon hot pepper sauce, such as Tabasco

Finely grated zest and juice of 1 lemon

4 scallions, finely chopped

1 cup (packed) baby spinach leaves, coarsely chopped

1 small red bell pepper, seeded and finely chopped

1 celery rib, finely chopped

Cucumber-Yogurt Sauce (recipe follows)

Preheat the oven to 425°F. Generously spray a 12-cup (2½-inch) cupcake or muffin tin with nonstick cooking spray.

Drain the salmon well. Flake and pick over to remove the skin and any unusually large bones. Mash the smaller bones, which are rich in calcium; they will dissolve when cooked.

In a food processor or blender, combine the bread and oats. Process, pulsing the machine on and off, to form crumbs.

In a large bowl, whisk the eggs with the salt until well blended. Whisk in the mayonnaise, mustard, and hot sauce. Stir in the lemon zest and juice and the oatmeal-crumb mixture. Add the scallions, spinach, bell pepper, and celery and mix well. Stir in the salmon. Divide the mixture evenly among the prepared cups, pressing down gently to fill.

Bake the salmon cakes until they are lightly browned on top and a knife inserted into the center shows no evidence of uncooked egg, 12 to 15 minutes. Let cool in the pan for 10 to 15 minutes, then use a blunt knife to ease the cakes out of the pan. Serve warm, at room temperature, or slightly chilled, topped with a generous dollop of Cucumber-Yogurt Sauce. Refrigerate leftover cakes for up to 2 days, or freeze for longer storage.

continued

Cucumber-Yogurt Sauce

MAKES ABOUT 1½ CUPS; 6 SERVINGS | 2 POINTS EACH

This sauce requires some time to drain the yogurt and develop its flavors, so begin a day ahead if you can.

8 ounces (1 cup) plain whole-milk yogurt, preferably goat's milk yogurt

½ English hothouse cucumber, halved lengthwise, seeded, and coarsely grated

1½ teaspoons coarse (kosher) salt

¼ cup full-fat sour cream

1 tablespoon freshly squeezed lemon juice

1 tablespoon finely chopped fresh dill or 1 teaspoon dried dill

1 small clove garlic, crushed through a press

⅛ teaspoon ground cumin

Freshly ground pepper

Line a sieve with cheesecloth, an unbleached coffee filter, or a double layer of white paper towels and place over a bowl. Spoon the yogurt into the lined sieve, cover with plastic wrap, and let drain in the refrigerator overnight.

In another bowl, toss the cucumber with the salt. Cover and refrigerate for 3 hours.

Transfer the drained yogurt to a clean bowl. (Discard the liquid whey or save it for soup stock.) Stir in the sour cream, lemon juice, dill, garlic, and cumin.

With your hands, squeeze out as much liquid as possible from the cucumber. Stir the cucumber into the yogurt mixture. Season to taste with pepper. Cover and refrigerate for at least 2 hours or up to 8 hours to blend the flavors before serving.

Spanish Garlic Shrimp

4 SERVINGS | 20 POINTS EACH

Here is one of the best ways to enjoy extra-virgin olive oil. Most supermarkets sell smoked paprika, but if you can get hold of some real Spanish bittersweet *pimento de la Vera,* you'll find it's a real treat.

1 pound large shrimp

2 tablespoons medium-dry sherry or dry white wine

Coarse sea salt and freshly ground pepper

⅓ cup extra-virgin olive oil

3 cloves garlic, thinly sliced

1 teaspoon smoked Spanish paprika

Shell and devein the shrimp, leaving the tail on, if desired. Toss the shrimp with the sherry and a pinch of sea salt and pepper and let stand for about 10 minutes. Remove the shrimp from the marinade and pat dry on paper towels.

In a large cast-iron skillet or wok, heat 3 tablespoons of the olive oil over high heat until very hot. Add the shrimp and garlic. Sauté, tossing, until the shrimp are pink and loosely curled, about 2 minutes.

Decrease the heat to medium. Sprinkle the smoked paprika, another pinch of salt, and the remaining 2⅓ tablespoons of olive oil over the shrimp and cook until they are opaque in the center, about 1 minute longer. Transfer to a serving platter and scrape the oil and garlic over the shrimp.

Tilapia in Tomato-Caper Sauce with Kalamata Olives

4 SERVINGS | 23 POINTS EACH

Here tender white fish fillets are essentially poached in a light tomato sauce, rich with Mediterranean flavors. You could do the same recipe with striped or black bass, cod, or even halibut.

20 ounces (1¼ pounds) tilapia fillets

Salt and freshly ground pepper

1 leek (white and tender green parts), thinly sliced

3 tablespoons extra-virgin olive oil

2 cloves garlic, finely chopped

1 tablespoon tiny (non-pareil) capers

½ cup dry white wine

1½ cups diced canned tomatoes with their juices

9 pitted kalamata olives, quartered lengthwise

⅛ teaspoon crushed hot red pepper, or more to taste

¼ cup coarsely chopped parsley

Pat the fish dry. Season on both side with salt and pepper. Refrigerate while you make the sauce.

In a large skillet, sauté the leek in the olive oil over medium heat until softened, about 3 minutes. Add the garlic and capers and cook until the garlic is fragrant, 1 to 2 minutes longer. Pour in the wine and bring to a boil. Boil until the liquid is reduced by about half, 1 to 2 minutes.

Add the tomatoes and olives, partially cover the skillet, and simmer for 5 minutes. Taste the sauce and season with additional salt, pepper, and hot red pepper as needed. Stir in 3 tablespoons of the parsley.

Add the fish fillets to the pan, spooning up the sauce to coat them. Cover, decrease the heat to medium-low, and simmer for 4 minutes. If the fillets are not submerged in the sauce, carefully turn them over with a spatula and simmer until the fish is 145°F in the center or no longer translucent and just beginning to flake, 3 to 4 minutes longer. Serve with the remaining 1 tablespoon of parsley sprinkled on top.

Tuscan Shrimp with Cranberry Beans

4 SERVINGS | 22 POINTS EACH

You don't need large shrimp for this recipe, but the fresher and sweeter they are, the better the flavor. Cranberry beans, known as *borlotti* beans in Italy, have a nice creamy consistency and lovely color, but cannellini, pink beans, or even pinto beans make a fine substitute.

1 pound shelled and deveined shrimp

Salt and freshly ground pepper

6 large sage leaves, slivered

5 tablespoons extra-virgin olive oil

3 cloves garlic, thinly sliced

1 cup chicken broth

2 cups cooked or canned cranberry beans (*borlotti*)

1 tablespoon freshly squeezed lemon juice

⅓ cup chopped fresh parsley

Season the shrimp with salt and pepper.

In a small skillet or saucepan, cook the slivered sage in 1 tablespoon of the olive oil over medium heat until they darken, about 2 minutes. Remove from the heat immediately and scrape them into a small bowl, saving as much of the oil as you can.

In a cast-iron skillet or wok, heat 2½ tablespoons of the olive oil over high heat until very hot. Toss in the shrimp and cook, stirring once or twice, until they are pink and curled, 1½ to 2 minutes. Transfer the shrimp to a plate; decrease the heat to medium.

Add the remaining 1½ tablespoons of olive oil and the garlic. Cook until the garlic is just beginning to color. Immediately pour in the broth. Add the beans, lemon juice, ¼ cup of the parsley, and the sautéed sage leaves with their oil. Bring to a simmer, mashing some of the beans to thicken the sauce, and cook for 5 minutes.

Return the shrimp to the pan, along with any juices that have collected on the plate. Season with additional salt and pepper to taste. Simmer for 2 minutes and serve with the remaining 1⅓ tablespoons of parsley sprinkled on top.

Mussels Steamed in White Wine with Herbs

4 SERVINGS | 19 POINTS EACH

Mussels are incredibly lean and require so much work to eat that you can take your time and fill up while still eating light. Start your meal with a nice green salad tossed with a variety of fresh vegetables of different colors, and, if you have the points, enjoy a slice of whole grain bread toasted and rubbed with garlic. You'll want to use a spoon to enjoy every drop of the flavorful juices.

4 pounds mussels, preferably farm raised (because they are cleaner)	3 tablespoons minced shallots	Pinch of crushed hot red pepper
	2 cloves garlic, minced	½ cup dry white wine or dry vermouth
3 tablespoons extra-virgin olive oil	¼ teaspoon dried thyme	¼ cup chopped parsley

Scrub the mussels well under cold running water. Tug on their hairy "beards" and cut them off with a small sharp knife.

In a large deep pot, warm the olive oil over medium heat. Add the shallots and cook to soften, 2 to 3 minutes. Add the garlic, thyme, and hot red pepper and cook 1 minute longer. Pour in the wine and add 3 tablespoons of the parsley. Raise the heat to high and bring to a rolling boil.

Dump in the mussels and immediately cover the pot. Steam for 3 to 5 minutes, or until the mussels just open. Remove with a slotted spoon or skimmer, dividing them among 4 soup plates.

If any of the mussels have not opened, boil them in the broth for another 2 minutes. If they are still closed, discard. Pour the hot broth over the mussels, avoiding any grit at the bottom of the pot. Sprinkle the remaining 1 tablespooon of parsley on top and serve at once.

Moroccan Fish Tagine en Papillote

4 SERVINGS | 17 POINTS EACH

Here are all the savory flavors of a fish tagine, wrapped up in individual packets. Present each guest with his or her own gift-wrapped entree that, when opened at the table, emits the heady aroma of Moroccan spices. Best of all, the dish can be prepared early in the day and refrigerated until baking time, perfect for easy entertaining. The same dish could also be done with salmon, snapper, or even tilapia, though the cooking time might vary slightly.

1 (15-ounce) can chickpeas (garbanzo beans), well rinsed and drained	1 carrot, finely chopped	½ teaspoon ground coriander
	1 shallot, finely chopped	½ teaspoon finely grated lemon zest
2 small ripe tomatoes, chopped	1½ tablespoons extra-virgin olive oil	Salt
1 red or yellow bell pepper, seeded and cut into ½-inch dice	2 teaspoons chopped flat-leaf parsley	¼ teaspoon crushed hot red pepper
2 zucchini, cut into ½-inch dice	1 clove garlic, crushed through a press	12 to 14 ounces skinless Arctic char fillets
1 celery rib, finely chopped	¾ teaspoon ground cumin	Freshly ground pepper

continued

Preheat the oven to 450°F. In a bowl, mix together the chickpeas, tomatoes, bell pepper, zucchini, celery, carrot, shallot, oil, parsley, garlic, cumin, coriander, lemon zest, ½ teaspoon salt, and hot red pepper.

Arrange 4 (16 by 12-inch) sheets of parchment paper (or nonstick aluminum foil, nonstick side up) on a work surface. Divide the fish into 4 equal pieces. Place one fish fillet in the center of each sheet and season lightly with salt and pepper. Place one-quarter of the chickpea and vegetable mixture over each fillet. Working one at a time, bring up the edges of the sheet over the fish and chickpea mixture, double-folding to form a tight seal and leaving room for heat circulation inside the packet. Use a metal spatula to transfer each packet to a baking sheet.

Bake for 18 to 20 minutes, or until the vegetables are tender and the fish is cooked through.

Spice-Rubbed Salmon Kebabs with Minted Yogurt Sauce

6 SERVINGS | 17 POINTS EACH

Grilled kebabs are an especially good technique for wild salmon, particularly lean coho. Look for the thickest center-cut salmon fillet to make nice-size chunks. If you prefer to use your barbecue, the smoke will add an extra note of flavor, but for simplicity, this recipe grills the kebabs under a very hot broiler. I like to serve this dish with chewy Wheat Berry Salad (page 210), which can be prepared earlier in the day. It would also go well with one of the quinoa salads or the Dilled Barley Salad with Corn and Edamame (page 208).

1½ pounds skinless, center-cut salmon fillet, cut into 1- to 1½-inch cubes or chunks

1 teaspoon ground cumin

1 teaspoon za'atar spice blend or dried thyme leaves

½ teaspoon smoked paprika

½ teaspoon salt

1 red bell pepper, seeded and cut into 1-inch cubes

12 scallions, trimmed bulb and 1 inch of pale green stalk

12 large white or cremini mushrooms

12 bamboo skewers, soaked in warm water for 1 hour to prevent burning

6 cups (lightly packed) baby arugula leaves

Minted Yogurt Sauce (recipe follows)

Position a rack 6 inches from the top of the oven. Preheat the broiler until hot. Cover a broiler pan or heavy baking sheet with foil, and spray with nonstick cooking spray.

Pat the salmon dry with paper towels. In a large bowl, mix together the cumin, za'atar, paprika, and salt. Add the salmon and toss gently to coat.

Thread 2 or 3 pieces of salmon and red pepper and 2 scallions and mushrooms onto each skewer, alternating the ingredients without crowding.

Arrange 2 rows of kebabs on the prepared broiler pan with all of the skewer "handles" facing out, allowing at least 1 inch between each one. Broil until the salmon is lightly browned on the outside and barely opaque in the center, 5 to 7 minutes.

To serve, mound 1 cup of arugula over the center of each plate and top with a couple of the salmon kebabs. Drizzle Minted Yogurt Sauce over the fish or pass on the side. Serve warm or at room temperature.

Minted Yogurt Sauce

MAKES ABOUT ⅔ CUP; 6 SERVINGS | ½ POINT EACH

Refreshing mint, zesty scallion, and lemon add zing to this simple, creamy sauce. We call for whole-milk yogurt because recent studies show that dairy fat may help to improve insulin resistance.

6 ounces (about ⅔ cup) plain whole-milk yogurt, preferably goat's milk yogurt	2 tablespoons chopped fresh mint 1 scallion, finely chopped	1 tablespoon freshly squeezed lemon juice ½ teaspoon salt ⅛ teaspoon cayenne pepper

In a bowl, stir together the yogurt, mint, scallion, lemon juice, salt, and cayenne. Cover and refrigerate. Just before serving, stir well.

POULTRY

Chicken and turkey predominate here, with one recipe for Cornish game hen. These light meats are much healthier for anyone with diabetes or a weight issue. With less fat than red meat (assuming you remove the skin), chicken and turkey offer great sources of protein at a fraction of the caloric price. But even so, it's still about portion control: 4 or 5 ounces at dinner, 3 or 4 ounces at lunch. From a culinary point of view, these birds are infinitely versatile, pairing well with flavors that include Italian, Mexican, French, and Thai. We recommend using organic free-range birds whenever possible.

Balsamic Chicken with Mushrooms and Sweet Red Pepper

4 SERVINGS | 22 POINTS EACH

Serve with lots of steamed kale, chard, or spinach and ½ cup per person of polenta, brown rice, or roasted potatoes.

4 skinless, boneless chicken breasts (about 5 ounces each) or 2 large breasts (8 to 10 ounces each), cut in half

10 ounces sliced baby bella (portobello) or white mushrooms

1 large red bell pepper (about 8 ounces), seeded and cut into large wedges

¾ cup chicken broth

3 tablespoons balsamic vinegar

2 tablespoons extra-virgin olive oil

2 teaspoons soy sauce

1 teaspoon minced fresh rosemary or crumbled dried

⅛ to ¼ teaspoon crushed hot red pepper, to taste

Preheat the oven to 400°F.

Put the chicken in a shallow baking dish. Scatter the mushrooms and bell pepper pieces around the chicken.

In a small bowl, mix together the broth, vinegar, olive oil, soy sauce, rosemary, and hot red pepper. Pour over the chicken and vegetables and toss to coat.

Cover with foil and bake for 15 minutes. Decrease the oven temperature to 375°F, remove the foil, stir, and bake uncovered for 15 to 20 minutes more, until the chicken is just cooked through but still moist.

Italian-Style Baked Chicken Breasts with Mushrooms and Peppers

4 SERVINGS | 19 POINTS EACH

Based on the classic Italian cacciatore, this modern version is made quickly and easily with skinless, boneless chicken breasts. Bell peppers, which are rich in vitamins A and C, boost the fiber and nutrition. Serve with lightly steamed broccoli and, if you have the points, half a baked potato, a boiled or roasted Yukon potato, or ½ cup small pasta like orzo. If you're short on points, opt for ½ cup quinoa or brown rice.

---

1 pound skinless boneless chicken breasts, preferably large

3 tablespoons extra-virgin olive oil

8 ounces white button mushrooms, quartered or halved

1 onion, chopped

3 cloves garlic, chopped

1 red bell pepper, seeded and cut into 1½- to 2-inch pieces

1 green bell pepper, seeded and cut into 1½ to 2-inch pieces

1 teaspoon dried oregano

¼ teaspoon crushed hot red pepper, or more to taste

1 tablespoon tomato paste

1 cup chicken broth

1 (14.5-ounce) can diced tomatoes with their juices

1 teaspoon sea salt

Trim any fat, gristle, or membrane from the chicken. Cut into 2-inch chunks.

In a large skillet, heat 1 tablespoon of the olive oil. Add the mushrooms and sauté over medium-high heat, stirring only occasionally, until they are lightly browned and start to squeak when you stir them, 3 to 4 minutes. Transfer to a small bowl.

Add the onion and remaining 2 tablespoons oil to the same skillet. Decrease the heat to medium and cook, stirring, until the onion softens and turns golden, about 5 minutes.

Add the garlic and bell peppers and cook for 3 minutes. Stir in the oregano and hot red pepper. Add the tomato paste and cook, stirring, for 1 minute longer. Pour in the broth and bring to a boil, stirring to mix in the tomato paste. Add the diced tomatoes and salt. Bring to a simmer, decrease the heat to low, and cook for 10 minutes.

Add the chunks of chicken, pushing them down into the sauce. Cover and simmer, stirring and turning the chicken once or twice, for about 15 minutes, until the chicken is just cooked through but still moist.

Green Chicken Chili with White Beans

6 SERVINGS | 18 POINTS EACH

A one-dish meal, this mild chili is good enough to serve for company. If you want more spice, add a minced jalapeño or two to the mix. Serve in bowls with spoons to scoop up all the luscious juices.

1½ pounds well-trimmed skinless, boneless chicken thighs

2 fresh poblano peppers

1 large onion, chopped

3 tablespoons extra-virgin olive oil

4 cloves garlic, finely chopped

4 ounces fresh tomatillos (3 or 4), husked and finely diced

2 teaspoons ground cumin

1 teaspoon dried oregano

1 teaspoon coarse (kosher) salt

6 cups shredded collards and/or kale

1½ cups chicken broth

1 (5-ounce can) diced green chiles (mild)

1 (15-ounce) can cannellini or Great Northern white beans, rinsed and drained

Preheat the broiler on high. Trim the chicken thighs to remove any bits of fat or heavy veins. Cut each thigh into 2 or 3 pieces.

Roast the poblano peppers on a baking sheet under the broiler, turning until they are charred all over, 5 to 7 minutes. Place in a paper bag and let steam for 5 to 10 minutes. Remove and rub off as much skin as possible. Cut the peppers into ½-inch dice.

In a flameproof casserole or large, deep skillet, cook the onion in the olive oil, covered, over low heat for 5 minutes. Uncover, raise the heat to medium-high, and sauté until golden and beginning to brown, 5 to 7 minutes longer. Add the garlic and tomatillos and cook for 2 minutes.

Add the chicken pieces, turning to coat with the oil. Season with the cumin, oregano, and salt. Cook, stirring, until the outside of the chicken is mostly white, 3 to 5 minutes. Stir in the greens. Add the broth and chiles.

Bring to a boil, decrease the heat to medium-low, partially cover, and simmer for 10 minutes. Add the beans and simmer for 5 minutes more.

Chicken with 40 Cloves of Garlic

6 SERVINGS | 22 POINTS EACH

If you've never had this classic French dish, you'll be amazed at how the garlic is transformed into a mild, sweet vegetable. The recipe calls for fairly small chicken thighs; if all you can find are large, simply buy fewer and cut in half. Serve with ½ cup of brown rice or orzo and a couple of lovely steamed vegetables, such as broccoli and carrots or green beans and sliced kohlrabi. A garnish of chopped parsley would really brighten up this dish.

6 chicken thighs (about 5 ounces each), skinned

⅓ cup all-purpose flour

Salt and freshly ground pepper

4 heads garlic

2 tablespoons extra-virgin olive oil

2 tablespoons unsalted butter

¾ teaspoon dried thyme

½ cup dry white wine or vermouth

1½ cups reduced-sodium chicken broth

Trim any excess fat from the chicken. Season the flour with 1 teaspoon of salt and ¼ teaspoon of pepper. Dust the chicken with the seasoned flour to coat all over. Shake off any excess.

Divide the garlic into separate cloves and peel. To speed up this task, put the whole heads inside 2 matching, stainless steel bowls and shake hard. Most of the cloves will separate and shed their skins.

Heat the olive oil in a large skillet over medium-high heat. Add the chicken and sauté, turning once, until golden brown on both sides, about 3 minutes per side. Pour out any excess fat. Decrease the heat to medium.

Add the butter and thyme and the peeled garlic cloves to the pan. Cook gently for 1 to 2 minutes without browning. Pour in the wine and bring to a boil. Boil for 1 full minute to reduce slightly and burn off some of the alcohol.

Pour the broth into the pan, cover, and simmer over medium-low heat, turning the thighs once or twice, for 45 to 50 minutes, or until the chicken is tender and the garlic is mellow and meltingly soft.

Remove the chicken and garlic to a deep platter or serving dish. If necessary, boil the liquid in the pan until it reduces and thickens slightly. Season with salt and pepper to taste, pour it over the chicken, and serve.

Savory Chicken and White Bean Bake

6 SERVINGS | 24 POINTS EACH

Chunks of skinless, boneless chicken thighs marinated for deep flavor make this hearty, high-fiber dish meaty and memorable. Because it can be prepared entirely in advance, it's perfect for company or for Sunday supper. Serve with steamed kale or sautéed brussels sprouts.

6 small or 5 large chicken thighs, 1½ to 1¾ pounds, trimmed of all fat and cut into 2-inch chunks

2 tablespoons freshly squeezed lemon juice

3 tablespoons extra-virgin olive oil

2 cloves garlic, crushed through a press

1½ teaspoons dried or fresh thyme

1 teaspoon dried rosemary

1 teaspoon salt

½ teaspoon freshly ground pepper

1 onion, chopped

4 carrots, peeled and diced

1 (14.5-ounce) can diced tomatoes

2¾ cups cooked or canned cannellini or Great Northern white beans, drained and rinsed

⅓ cup Italian seasoned bread crumbs

Several hours in advance or the night before, toss the chicken chunks with the lemon juice, 1½ teaspoons of the olive oil, 1 of the crushed garlic cloves, 1 teaspoon of the thyme, ½ teaspoon of the rosemary, ½ teaspoon of the salt, and ¼ teaspoon of the pepper. Cover and refrigerate for at least 3 hours or overnight.

In a large enameled paella pan or flameproof casserole, heat 2 tablespoons of the olive oil. Add the onion and carrots and sauté over medium-high heat, stirring occasionally, until the onion is golden and beginning to brown, about 5 minutes.

Add the chicken with its marinade. Continue to cook, stirring occasionally, until the meat loses its pink color, 3 to 5 minutes. Add the tomatoes, the remaining clove of crushed garlic, the remaining ½ teaspoon each of thyme and rosemary, the remaining ½ teaspoon of salt, and the remaining ¼ teaspoon of pepper. Decrease the heat to medium-low, cover, and simmer for 10 minutes, turning the chicken once or twice.

Add the beans, mashing some of them into the sauce. Continue to simmer, uncovered, until the chicken is just cooked through and the sauce is beginning to thicken, about 10 minutes longer. (The recipe can be made up to this point up to 2 days in advance. If not serving, let cool slightly, then cover and refrigerate. When ready to complete the dish, let stand at room temperature for about an hour before proceeding.)

About 30 minutes before you plan on serving, preheat the oven to 375°F. Sprinkle the bread crumbs over the top of the casserole and drizzle with the remaining 1½ teaspoons olive oil. Bake until the casserole is bubbly, 15 to 20 minutes. Run under the broiler for 3 to 5 minutes to brown the top lightly.

Stuffed Turkey Breast

6 SERVINGS | 24 POINTS EACH

Here is a festive dish that will brighten any dinner table. You can do it all in one fell swoop, or prepare the rolled turkey a day ahead and cook it shortly before serving. Serve with quinoa or roasted potatoes and offer another vegetable, such as sautéed broccoli rabe or Lemony Stir-Fried Brussels Sprouts (page 204).

1¾ pounds turkey breast

Salt and freshly ground pepper

½ cup finely chopped onion

1½ tablespoons olive oil

10 ounces frozen chopped spinach, thawed and squeezed dry

¼ teaspoon freshly grated nutmeg

2½ ounces thinly sliced provolone

2 or 3 paper-thin slices prosciutto, turkey bacon, or speck

½ cup dry white wine

¾ cup reduced-sodium chicken stock

Preheat the oven to 325°F. If the turkey is on the bone, remove the skin and bone. If it is a fillet, also remove any skin. Trim off any excess fat. Pound the meat gently to flatten as evenly as possible. Season lightly with salt and pepper.

In a skillet, cook the onion in the olive oil over medium heat until soft and just beginning to turn golden, 5 to 7 minutes. Stir in the spinach and heat through. Season with the nutmeg, ¼ teaspoon of salt, and a generous grinding of pepper.

Arrange the provolone over the turkey to cover it in a single layer. Spoon the spinach mixture down the length of the turkey and squeeze the mixture together with your hands to form a log in the center. Roll up the turkey to enclose the spinach. Fasten the turkey closed with toothpicks or poultry skewers. Wrap the outside with the prosciutto. Tie with string so the roast will keep its nice shape.

Place in a small roasting pan or gratin dish and add the wine and stock; cover the pan with foil. Roast the turkey for 45 minutes, then uncover and roast for 20 minutes longer, or until the turkey registers 160°F on an instant-read thermometer. Remove the pan from the oven, tent with foil, and let stand for 5 to 10 minutes longer to finish cooking.

Remove the string and fasteners and carve into ½-inch slices.

Turkey Scaloppine with Garlic and Cherry Peppers

4 SERVINGS | 22 POINTS EACH

Scaloppine is traditionally made with pork. In this version with turkey, which is chameleon-like, taking on the character and flavor of its sauce, the piquant cherry peppers, tart vinegar, and aromatic garlic work beautifully to add interest to the dish. Serve with brown rice, roasted potatoes, or a small serving of pasta and be sure to include a couple of steamed vegetables, such as kale and zucchini.

1 pound turkey breast, cut into ¼-inch-thick slices	⅛ teaspoon freshly ground pepper	5 sprigs fresh rosemary or ½ teaspoon dried
⅓ cup all-purpose flour	3 tablespoons extra-virgin olive oil	⅓ cup dry white wine
½ teaspoon dried thyme	5 cloves garlic, smashed	⅔ cup chicken broth
½ teaspoon salt	3 sweet-hot cherry peppers (jarred in brine)	3 tablespoons red wine vinegar or sherry vinegar

Trim any fat or gristle from the turkey. On a large plate, mix the flour with the thyme, salt, and pepper. Dredge the turkey in the seasoned flour to coat all over. Shake off any excess.

Heat the olive oil in a large skillet over medium-high heat. Add the turkey and sauté briefly, turning to brown lightly, about 2 minutes per side.

Add the garlic, cherry peppers, rosemary, and wine. Boil for 1 to 2 minutes to reduce the wine slightly. Add the broth and vinegar. Decrease the heat to medium-low, cover, and simmer, stirring occasionally, until the turkey is tender, 15 to 20 minutes.

Turkey Piccata

4 SERVINGS | 25 POINTS EACH

Turkey is higher in iron than chicken and mild enough to substitute for veal, which is not available in many markets. Either buy thinly sliced turkey breast or partially freeze the whole breast, then cut across the grain on a slight diagonal.

1 pound thinly sliced turkey breast	3½ tablespoons extra-virgin olive oil	1 to 2 teaspoons grated lemon zest
½ cup all-purpose flour	1 large shallot, minced	2 tablespoons freshly squeezed lemon juice
½ teaspoon salt	⅓ cup dry white wine	
⅛ teaspoon freshly ground pepper	⅓ cup chicken broth	1 to 2 tablespoons tiny (nonpareil) capers

Place the turkey slices between 2 slices of waxed paper and pound gently to thin evenly. Spread out the flour on a plate. Season with the salt and pepper. Dredge the turkey slices in the seasoned flour; shake off any excess.

Heat 2 tablespoons of the oil in a large skillet over medium heat. Add the turkey cutlets and cook until lightly browned outside and cooked through, 2 to 3 minutes on each side. Set aside on a platter or plates.

Pour out the oil and discard; wipe out the pan. Heat the remaining 1½ tablespoons oil with the shallot over medium heat. Cook until the shallot is soft and fragrant, 1 to 2 minutes. Pour in the wine and boil until reduced to a couple of tablespoons. Pour in the chicken broth, lemon zest, lemon juice, and capers and cook until heated through. Pour over the turkey and serve.

Asian Turkey Meatball Wraps

MAKES ABOUT 18 MEATBALLS; 6 SERVINGS | 17 POINTS EACH

Although you could opt to serve these flavor-packed meatballs in a whole wheat pita pocket, we prefer the lighter option of wrapping them in tender lettuce leaves. Set out all the fillings on a platter so your guests can custom design their own wrap.

⅓ cup bulgur	3 tablespoons soy sauce	About 1 tablespoon sunflower oil, or as needed
2 heads butter lettuce (also known as Boston lettuce or Bibb lettuce)	2 teaspoons Sriracha or other hot-pepper sauce, plus more for serving	2 tomatoes, chopped
1½ pounds ground turkey	2 teaspoons Asian sesame oil	1 small cucumber, thinly sliced
3 scallions, chopped	2 cloves garlic, crushed through a press	½ small red onion, thinly sliced
1 carrot, grated	1 teaspoon salt	18 small sprigs cilantro
1 egg, lightly beaten		Lime wedges, for serving

In a bowl, combine the bulgur with enough hot water to cover by 1 inch. Let stand for 10 minutes to soften. Drain well in a fine sieve.

Preheat the oven to 450°F. Break apart the heads of lettuce, pulling back the leaves to separate. Refrigerate 18 of the small, tender leaves to use as cups for the meatballs. Reserve the outer leaves for salads or another use.

In a bowl, combine the bulgur, turkey, scallions, carrot, egg, soy sauce, Sriracha, sesame oil, garlic, and salt. Form into 18 meatballs, each about 1½ inches in diameter.

continued

Asian Turkey Meatball Wraps, continued

In a large nonstick skillet, heat 2 teaspoons of the sunflower oil over medium-high heat. Working in batches, cook the meatballs without crowding, turning often to brown all over, about 10 minutes. As each batch is browned, transfer to a baking sheet. Continue to cook the remaining meatballs in batches, adding more oil to the pan if needed.

Bake the browned meatballs, shaking the pan once or twice to cook evenly, until the turkey is white throughout, about 10 minutes. Let cool for 5 minutes.

To serve, place 1 warm meatball in a lettuce cup, along with a spoonful of chopped tomatoes, a few slices of cucumber and onion, and a cilantro sprig. Pass the Sriracha sauce and lime wedges to squeeze over the filling. Fold the lettuce over the filling and eat as you would a taco.

Five-Spice Cornish Game Hens with Thai Confetti Slaw

4 SERVINGS | 21 POINTS EACH

A crispy-skinned game hen makes an appealing entree any time of year, especially when served atop crunchy coleslaw dotted with chunks of fresh pineapple. Use poultry shears to cut the hens in half, or ask your butcher to do it for you. When planning the preparation, allow for the advance time needed to marinate the hens.

2 Cornish game hens (about 1 pound each)

2 large cloves garlic, crushed through a press or finely chopped

2 teaspoons sunflower oil

2 teaspoons light brown sugar

2 teaspoons Asian fish sauce (Thai *nam pla* or Vietnamese *nuoc mam*)

2 teaspoons freshly squeezed lime juice

½ teaspoon Chinese five-spice powder

¼ teaspoon salt

Dash of cayenne pepper

Thai Confetti Slaw (recipe follows)

2 scallions, thinly sliced on the diagonal

1½ teaspoons toasted sesame seeds

Halve each hen by cutting through the breast and the backbone. Using the palm of your hand, press down firmly on each breast to flatten. Pat dry with paper towels.

In a small bowl, combine the garlic, oil, sugar, fish sauce, lime juice, five-spice powder, salt, and cayenne. Stir, mashing the ingredients to form a paste. Rub the mixture all over the hens and marinate at room temperature for 1 to 2 hours, or overnight in the refrigerator. (If chilled, return to room temperature before cooking.)

Position a rack in the upper third of the oven and preheat to 450°F.

Spray a broiler pan or heavy rimmed baking sheet with nonstick cooking spray and arrange the hen halves cut side down. Bake until the skin is nicely browned and an instant-read thermometer inserted into the meatiest part of the thigh (without touching the bone) registers 165°F, 25 to 30 minutes. Let stand for 5 to 10 minutes before serving.

Divide the slaw among 4 plates and top each with a half hen. Sprinkle the scallion slices and sesame seeds over all.

Thai Confetti Slaw

4 SERVINGS | 3 POINTS EACH

Light, fresh, and crisp, this easy cabbage salad can be whipped up in minutes by using a large sharp knife or the slicing blade in a food processor to shred the cabbage. Fresh pineapple adds a sweet-tart note that provides a perfect counterpoint to the salty fish sauce. Serve with grilled chicken or shrimp.

2 tablespoons freshly squeezed lime juice

2 tablespoons unseasoned rice vinegar

1 teaspoon Asian fish sauce (Thai *nam pla* or Vietnamese *nuoc mam*)

1 teaspoon light brown sugar

2 tablespoons sunflower oil

1 teaspoon grated fresh ginger

6 cups very thinly sliced green cabbage (about ½ head)

½ fresh pineapple, peeled, cored, and cut into ½-inch chunks

1 small red bell pepper, seeded and cut into ¼-inch dice or chopped

1 carrot, grated

⅓ cup coarsely chopped fresh cilantro and/or mint

In a large bowl, mix together the lime juice, vinegar, fish sauce, and sugar. Add 1 tablespoon of water and the oil, whisking until blended. Stir in the ginger. Add the cabbage, pineapple, bell pepper, and carrot and toss gently to coat. Cover and refrigerate for at least 30 minutes to let the flavors blend. Just before serving, stir in the cilantro and/or mint.

Joe's Special One-Skillet Meal

4 SERVINGS | 13 POINTS EACH

Joe's Special is arguably the most famous one-skillet dish in the Bay Area, harking back to the days when San Francisco was known for its rough Barbary Coast. Originally intended as an antidote for late-night revelry, it's now a popular choice for breakfast, lunch, and dinner. Here it's given a twenty-first-century makeover with lean ground turkey instead of beef, plus the addition of some other California favorites: mushrooms, artichokes, and sun-dried tomatoes. If you are a devotee of all things spicy, by all means pass the Tabasco or other favorite hot sauce at the table.

continued

2 tablespoons extra-virgin olive oil

1 onion, chopped

4 ounces mushrooms, sliced

1 clove garlic, finely chopped

8 ounces ground turkey

½ teaspoon Italian seasoning blend

¾ teaspoon salt

Freshly ground pepper, to taste

8 frozen artichoke heart halves, thawed and cut in half lengthwise

4 cups baby spinach leaves (about 3 ounces)

2 oil-packed sun-dried tomato halves, finely chopped (about 2 tablespoons)

4 large eggs, lightly beaten

2 tablespoons freshly grated Parmesan cheese

In a 12-inch skillet (preferably nonstick), heat the oil over medium heat. Add the onion, mushrooms, and garlic and cook, stirring occasionally, until the onion has softened but not browned, 4 to 5 minutes.

Add the turkey, Italian seasoning, salt, and pepper. Cook, breaking up the meat with a heatproof spatula or wooden spoon, until the turkey is white throughout, about 5 minutes.

Stir in the artichoke hearts and cook for 2 minutes longer. Add the spinach and sun-dried tomatoes, stirring until the spinach wilts, 1 to 2 minutes. Add the eggs, stirring until set, about 2 minutes. Sprinkle 1½ teaspoons of the cheese over each serving.

RED MEATS: BEEF, PORK, LAMB

Red meat in quantity is never a good choice for diabetes or weight control, but lean cuts in small amounts eaten occasionally offer culinary variety and valuable nutrients. Vitamin A, B12, iron, and zinc are just some of the hard-to-obtain nutrients packed into red meat.

Steak Fajitas

4 SERVINGS | 18 POINTS EACH

Red meat should be a treat rather than an everyday staple, but when you crave it, the flavor should be over the top. Here's a dynamite dish that offers an appropriate 3 ounces of meat paired with a whopping 7 grams of dietary fiber. Serve with a crisp green salad or slaw seasoned with lime, and ½ cup brown rice or corn.

2 rib steaks, well trimmed (about 6 ounces each)	1 tablespoon extra-virgin olive oil	1 teaspoon dried marjoram (see Note)
Sea salt and freshly ground pepper	2 teaspoons Worcestershire sauce	4 (8-inch) whole wheat tortillas
3 tablespoons freshly squeezed lime juice	3 cloves garlic, crushed through a press	¾ cup fat-free refried beans
1 tablespoon soy sauce	1 shallot, minced	Rajas (recipe follows)

Trim off any fat rimming the steaks or any big chunks in the middle. Season generously on both sides with salt and pepper.

In a glass pie plate or shallow baking dish, mix the lime juice, soy sauce, oil, Worcestershire, garlic, shallot, and marjoram. Add the steaks and turn to coat both sides. Marinate at room temperature for 30 to 60 minutes or in the refrigerator for up to 6 hours, turning occasionally.

Light a hot fire in a barbecue grill or heat a stove-top grill pan until hot. Grill the steaks until medium-rare, 3 to 4 minutes per side, or longer if you prefer your meat well done. Remove to a cutting board and let rest, covered loosely with foil, for 3 to 5 minutes. Heat the tortillas briefly until softened on the grill or in a warm oven.

Carve the steak crosswise into strips. Serve with the tortillas, refried beans, and rajas.

Note: If you don't have marjoram in the house you can substitute ½ teaspoon each dried thyme and oregano.

continued

Rajas

4 TO 6 SERVINGS | 2 TO 3 POINTS EACH

Rajas is a traditional Mexican accompaniment to grilled meats and tortilla dishes. Usually made simply with poblano peppers, this version brightens things up with a red bell pepper as well.

1 large or 2 medium poblano peppers	2 tablespoons extra-virgin olive oil	½ teaspoon cumin seeds, crushed
1 red bell pepper	1 white onion, cut into rounds	Pinch of salt

Char the poblano and bell peppers on a hot grill, over an open gas flame, or on a baking sheet under the broiler, turning until the peppers are blackened all over. Place the charred peppers in a paper bag and let steam for 5 minutes; remove and rub off as much skin as possible. Stem and seed the peppers, then cut them into strips.

In a large skillet, heat the olive oil over high heat until very hot. Add the onion and sauté until slightly softened and browned at the edges, 2 to 3 minutes. Add the cumin and cook for 30 seconds; add the peppers and sauté until heated through, 1 to 2 minutes more. Season lightly with salt.

Thai Grilled Beef Salad

4 SERVINGS | 11 POINTS EACH

Many Asian salads, such as this one, are very light on oil and high on taste. For extra color, garnish with wedges of ripe red tomato.

½ pound flank steak	2 teaspoons grated fresh ginger	½ cup coarsely chopped fresh cilantro
2 tablespoons soy sauce	2 cloves garlic, crushed through a press	1 tablespoon rice vinegar
1 tablespoon plus 2 teaspoons freshly squeezed lime juice	4 cups coarsely shredded green cabbage (about ½ head)	2 teaspoons Asian fish sauce
1 tablespoon peanut or canola oil	1 cup seeded and coarsely shredded red bell pepper	3 tablespoons coarsely chopped roasted peanuts
2 tablespoons cold water	2 carrots, coarsely shredded	2 tablespoons chopped scallions

Trim any outer fat from the steak. Place the meat in a glass pie plate. Pour the soy sauce, 1 tablespoon of the lime juice, the oil, and the cold water over the steak. Add 1 teaspoon of the ginger and the crushed garlic. Turn to coat on both sides. Set aside to marinate for at least 2 hours or up to 8 hours in the refrigerator.

Toss the cabbage, bell pepper, carrots, and cilantro with the vinegar, fish sauce, and the remaining 2 teaspoons of lime juice and 1 teaspoon of ginger. Cover and refrigerate to chill slightly.

Light a hot fire in a barbecue grill or preheat your broiler. Remove the meat from the marinade and pat dry. Grill, rotating and turning to make crisscross browned marks, until the meat is rare or medium-rare, 3 to 4 minute per side; if you over-cook it, the meat will be tough because it has so little fat. Transfer to a cutting board, cover loosely with foil, and let stand for 2 to 3 minutes. Then carve the meat against the grain on a slight angle into thin slices.

Make a bed of the cabbage salad on a deep platter or wide bowl. Arrange the grilled steak on top. Garnish with the chopped peanuts and scallions.

Mustard-Crusted Pork Tenderloin with Roasted Cabbage and Fennel

5 SERVINGS | 23 POINTS EACH

Don't be put off by the long ingredient list. This dish is easy and quick to make. Serve with wild rice, boiled Yukon gold potatoes, or baked sweet potato.

1 head green cabbage (1½ pounds), cored and cut into 1½-inch chunks	2 tablespoons dried cranberries	2 tablespoons quick-cooking or old-fashioned rolled oats
2 large fennel bulbs, halved and cut into ½-inch wedges	1½ teaspoons dried thyme	1 pork tenderloin (1 to 1¼ pounds), trimmed of any visible fat and silver skin
2 leeks (white and pale green parts), split lengthwise, sliced, and well rinsed	1½ tablespoons extra-virgin olive oil	
	Salt and freshly ground pepper	2 tablespoons Dijon mustard
2 carrots, peeled and sliced	½ cup chicken broth	1 teaspoon dried fennel seeds, crushed
	1 slice 100 percent whole wheat bread, torn into pieces (about 1 ounce)	1 clove garlic, crushed through a press

Preheat the oven to 450°F. In a shallow roasting pan or half-sheet pan, combine the cabbage, fennel, leeks, carrot, dried cranberries, ½ teaspoon of the thyme, the olive oil, 1 teaspoon of salt, and ¼ teaspoon of pepper. Toss gently to mix, then spread into an even layer. Drizzle the broth over all.

continued

In a food processor or blender, combine the bread and oatmeal. Process to form coarse crumbs. Add the remaining 1 teaspoon thyme and process, pulsing the machine on and off, until the herbs are well incorporated.

Season the pork with salt and pepper. In a small bowl, combine the mustard, fennel seeds, and garlic. Rub all over the pork, then roll it in the herbed bread crumbs to coat. Place the pork in the center of the pan, on top of the cabbage mixture. If needed, tuck the ends underneath the tenderloin so the meat is the same thickness throughout.

Bake, stirring the vegetable mixture around the pork once or twice, until an instant-read thermometer inserted into the center of the pork registers 150°F to 155°F, the fennel is crisp-tender, and the vegetables are lightly browned at the edges, 30 to 40 minutes. Transfer the pork to a cutting board to rest for 5 minutes before cutting into ½-inch-thick slices. Spread the vegetables onto a warm serving platter. Arrange the sliced pork on top and serve.

Hungarian Pork and Sauerkraut Goulash

6 SERVINGS | 26 POINTS EACH

Sauerkraut, like yogurt, is a natural probiotic; it also contains vitamins C and K and lots of fiber. This traditional stew is not only scrumptions, but it's also a good choice for a healthy meal. Serve with one or two small boiled or steamed Yukon gold potatoes, 2 ounces egg noodles, or a single slice of rye bread. Pass a small bowl of sour cream on the side.

2 pounds boneless pork loin, cut into 1-inch cubes	3 tablespoons imported Hungarian sweet paprika	¾ teaspoon dried thyme
Salt and freshly ground pepper	2 large sweet onions, sliced	⅛ to ¼ teaspoon cayenne pepper, to taste
2 tablespoons extra-virgin olive oil	½ cup dry white wine	½ cup full-fat sour cream, plus more for serving
	2 pounds sauerkraut	
	1½ cups chicken broth	

Season the pork with salt and pepper. In a large flameproof casserole, sauté the pork in the olive oil over medium-high heat until lightly browned all over, about 5 minutes. With a slotted spoon, transfer the meat to a bowl and toss with 1 tablespoon of the paprika.

Add the onions to the pot and cook, stirring, until softened, 5 to 7 minutes. Sprinkle on the remaining 2 tablespoons paprika and cook, stirring, for 1 minute.

Pour in the wine and bring to a boil; boil for 1 minute. Add the sauerkraut to the pot along with the broth, thyme, and cayenne pepper. Return to a boil, decrease the heat to low, and simmer, partially covered, for 1½ hours.

Stir in the sour cream and just heat through but do not boil. Season with additional salt and pepper to taste.

Middle Eastern Lamb and Eggplant Stew with Chickpeas and Tomatoes

4 SERVINGS | 17 POINTS EACH

This one-dish meal and the lamb curry, which follows, both offer good examples of how much food you can eat if a goodly proportion of it is composed of vegetables.

---

1 large Italian eggplant

Coarse salt

5 tablespoons extra-virgin olive oil

1 large onion, chopped

10 ounces boneless leg of lamb steak, trimmed and cut into ½-inch cubes

1 teaspoon ground cinnamon

½ teaspoon ground allspice

¼ teaspoon ground ginger

⅛ teaspoon freshly ground pepper

2 cups chopped canned tomatoes with their juices

1½ tablespoons freshly squeezed lemon juice

1 tablespoon pomegranate molasses

1 tablespoon harissa

1 cup cooked or canned chickpeas

Trim the eggplant and remove the peel from 2 sides. Cut the eggplant lengthwise into ½-inch-thick slices. Salt lightly on both sides and set in a colander to drain for 20 minutes or so. Then pat dry, pressing with paper towels to remove as much moisture as possible.

Preheat the broiler. Brush the eggplant on both sides with about 1½ tablespoons of the olive oil, place on a baking sheet, and broil, turning once, until browned and tender, 4 to 5 minutes per side. Transfer to a cutting board. When cool enough to handle, cut into ½-inch cubes.

In a large flameproof casserole or deep skillet, sauté the onion in the remaining 3½ tablespoons of olive oil over medium-high heat until softened and just beginning to color, about 5 minutes.

Add the lamb and sauté, stirring occasionally, until browned on the outside, 3 to 5 minutes. Add the cinnamon, allspice, ginger, and pepper. Toast the spices, stirring, for 1 minute.

Add the tomatoes, lemon juice, pomegranate molasses, and harissa. Bring to a boil, decrease the heat, and simmer, partially covered, for 30 minutes. Add the eggplant and chickpeas and simmer for 10 minutes longer. Season the sauce with additional salt and pepper to taste before serving.

Lamb and Vegetable Curry

4 SERVINGS | 15 POINTS EACH

We recommend eating only modest amounts of red meat, so pairing that meat with lots of vegetables, as in this curry, makes good sense in terms of portion size. The mix of spices creates a subtle and interesting flavor. Serve with ½ cup couscous or brown rice. If you like, pass a bowl of yogurt mixed with chopped cucumbers on the side.

---

12 ounces lean leg of lamb steak, cut ¾ inch thick

1 onion, cut into 6 wedges

1½ inches fresh ginger, peeled and sliced

3 cloves garlic

3 tablespoons extra-virgin olive oil

2 teaspoons ground coriander

1½ teaspoons ground cumin

1 teaspoon ground cinnamon

1 teaspoon salt

½ teaspoon crushed hot red pepper

1 cup chopped tomatoes

4 long, narrow Asian eggplants (about 1 pound)

¾ cup cut green beans

1 large red bell pepper, seeded and cut into 1½-inch pieces

Trim the lamb of all outer fat. Cut the meat into ¾-inch cubes.

Put the onion, ginger, and garlic in a blender or food processor and puree until finely chopped.

In a large flameproof casserole, sauté the ground onion mixture in the olive oil over medium-high heat until golden, 4 to 5 minutes. Add the lamb and season with the coriander, cumin, cinnamon, salt, and hot red pepper. Sauté, stirring often, to brown lightly, 2 to 3 minutes.

Pour in 2 cups of water and bring to a boil. Decrease the heat to low, cover, and simmer for 10 minutes. Add the tomatoes, eggplants, green beans, and bell pepper and continue to cook, covered, for 15 to 20 minutes, or until the lamb and vegetables are tender.

VEGETABLES AND BEANS

Vegetables in a variety of colors, raw and lightly cooked, and beans in modest portions should form the base of your glucose-lowering diet. When combined with healthy oils, they contribute a range of vitamins, minerals, and fibers that nourish your gut for optimum metabolism.

Asian Slaw

6 SERVINGS | 2 POINTS EACH

This is a sturdy slaw that holds up well in the refrigerator.

1 cup snow peas, trimmed	½ cup thinly sliced red cabbage	⅓ cup slivered scallions
1 cup thinly sliced napa cabbage	½ cup shredded carrot	Sesame-Ginger Dressing (recipe follows)
1 cup pea sprouts or bean sprouts	½ cup seeded and thinly sliced yellow bell pepper	2 tablespoons chopped cashews or peanuts

Bring a saucepan of salted water to a boil over high heat. Drop in the snow peas and cook until bright green, 10 to 15 seconds; drain. Rinse under cold running water and drain well. Cut the snow peas lengthwise into thin slivers.

Put the slivered snow peas into a salad bowl. Add the napa cabbage, pea sprouts, red cabbage, carrot, bell pepper, and scallions.

Shortly before serving, pour the dressing over the salad and toss to coat. Sprinkle the cashews over the salad and serve.

Sesame-Ginger Dressing

MAKES ABOUT ½ CUP; 6 SERVINGS | 1½ POINTS EACH

The combination of soy sauce, ginger, sesame oil, and garlic create an Asian-style dressing for this crisp slaw.

2 tablespoons peanut or extra-virgin olive oil	2 tablespoons soy sauce	2 tablespoons rice vinegar
2 tablespoons shredded fresh ginger	1 tablespoon light mirin	1 teaspoon toasted sesame oil
2 cloves garlic, minced	1 teaspoon brown sugar	

continued

...eat the oil in a small saucepan. Add the ginger and garlic and cook over medium heat until the garlic is softened and just beginning to turn golden, about 3 minutes.

Immediately pour in the soy sauce, mirin, and 1 tablespoon of water. Add the brown sugar and stir to dissolve. Simmer over low heat for 3 to 5 minutes. Remove from the heat and let cool.

Whisk in the vinegar and sesame oil.

Black Bean Tacquitos

6 SERVINGS | 7 POINTS EACH

You will not miss the meat with these mouthwatering bites of contrasting flavors and textures. They're a little like individual Mexican pizzas piled high with tasty ingredients, and the beans combined with the wheat provide complete protein that beans alone do not.

Jalapeño Cabbage Salad (recipe follows)	1 cup finely diced tomato	4 ounces Monterey Jack or Cheddar cheese, shredded (about 1¼ cups)
6 (8-inch) whole wheat tortillas	1 (15-ounce) can black beans, rinsed and well drained	½ cup Lemon Cream (page 162)
2 to 3 teaspoons extra-virgin olive oil	½ cup prepared tomato salsa	

Preheat the oven to 350°F. Prepare the cabbage salad and refrigerate.

Brush the tortillas lightly with the oil, place on a baking sheet, and bake until crisp, 5 to 7 minutes.

Toss together the diced tomato and black beans.

Divide the cabbage salad among the tortillas. Top with the tomato and beans. Spoon about 1½ tablespoons salsa over each, then sprinkle on about 3 tablespoons shredded cheese. Finally top each with about 1½ tablespoons of the lemon cream.

VARIATION: CHICKEN TACQUITOS (10 points per serving)
Prepare the Black Bean Tacquitos as directed, but decrease the black beans to 3 tablespoons on each tacquito and add 6 ounces of shredded roasted or rotisserie chicken (about ¼ cup on each).

Jalapeño Cabbage Salad

4 TO 6 SERVINGS | FREE

Refreshing and crisp, this slaw contains no oil and is best served fresh. Taste your chile before you add it, because heat levels can vary wildly. You can always add half and then a little more if you think it needs it.

½ head green cabbage, finely shredded (about 4 cups)

¾ teaspoon salt

3 tablespoons rice vinegar

1½ tablespoons freshly squeezed lime juice

1 jalapeño or serrano chile pepper, seeded and finely minced

Toss the cabbage with the salt. Add the vinegar, lime juice, and chile and mix well. Let stand for at least 5 to 10 minutes before serving.

Middle Eastern Chopped Salad

6 SERVINGS | FREE

This light salad, which contains no oil, is a traditional accompaniment to *ful medames* (page 155). Drained for a few minutes, it can be stirred into yogurt. Call it salsa and use it to dress grilled chicken or fish. Toss in some cooked shrimp for a light luncheon dish.

2 large beefsteak tomatoes, finely diced

1 teaspoon coarse (kosher) salt

2 small Persian cucumbers or ½ seedless English cucumber, finely diced

1 red bell pepper, seeded and finely diced

½ jalapeño or serrano pepper, seeded and minced

¼ cup finely diced red onion

¼ cup chopped cilantro or parsley

1 tablespoon red wine vinegar

2 teaspoons freshly squeezed lime or lemon juice

Toss the tomatoes with the salt and let drain in a sieve for 10 minutes. Transfer to a bowl. Add the cucumbers, peppers, red onion, and cilantro. Toss to mix. Dress with the vinegar and lime juice.

Broccoli Soufflé

6 SERVINGS AS A SIDE DISH, 4 AS A MAIN COURSE | 9 OR 13 POINTS EACH

Because this soufflé is prepared free-form, you don't have to worry about a special dish or collar, and it won't fall. It's not that high to begin with, but it's creamy, light, and fluffy. Serve as a vegetarian main course, with a green salad and tomatoes, or offer as a first course or side dish with roasted chicken or baked salmon.

4 tablespoons unsalted butter

¼ cup grated imported Parmesan cheese

1 pound broccoli

3 tablespoons all-purpose flour

1 cup hot whole milk

1 teaspoon salt

¼ teaspoon freshly grated nutmeg

Dash of cayenne pepper, or more to taste

6 eggs, separated

1½ cups coarsely grated imported Gruyère, Swiss, or Cheddar cheese

Preheat the oven to 425°F. Use 1½ teaspoons of the butter to grease a 14-inch oval gratin or 12-inch round baking dish. Sprinkle 2 tablespoons the grated Parmesan around the bottom and sides of the dish.

Peel the thick stems of the broccoli and cut into 1-inch pieces; separate the florets. Steam the stems and florets over boiling water until bright green and just barely tender, about 3 minutes. Rinse under cold running water. Coarsely chop the stems; cut the florets into ½-inch pieces.

In a saucepan, melt 3 tablespoons of the butter over medium heat. Add the flour and cook, stirring, for 2 minutes without allowing it to color. Gradually whisk in the hot milk. Bring to a boil, whisking, until the liquid thickens. Decrease the heat to low and simmer for 2 to 3 minutes longer. Season with the salt, nutmeg, and cayenne.

In a small bowl, beat the egg yolks. Gradually whisk ½ cup of the hot sauce into the yolks. Whisk the warmed yolks back into the remaining sauce. Remove from the heat and stir in the Gruyère cheese. When it is completely melted, stir in the broccoli stems and florets.

In a large bowl, whip the egg whites with a pinch of salt until stiff but not dry; err on the side of underbeating. If the whites are too stiff, the soufflé will deflate when it cooks. Fold one-fourth of the beaten egg whites into the broccoli mixture. Gently scrape the broccoli mixture over the remaining whites and fold with a rubber spatula until just mixed.

Turn the soufflé mixture into the prepared baking dish. Sprinkle the remaining 2 tablespoons of Parmesan cheese on top and dot with the remaining 1½ teaspoons butter. Bake for 25 minutes, or until the soufflé is puffed and the top is a lovely golden brown. Serve at once.

Eggplant Romano with Basil, Olives, and Sun-Dried Tomatoes

Balance the bright, salty flavors of this dish with a small serving of pasta or polenta. That means 2 ounces pasta (before cooking) or ½ cup cooked polenta. And be sure to include a generous side of steamed kale, Swiss chard, or broccoli rabe, plain or dressed with a drizzle of olive oil and lemon juice.

---

2 eggplants (¾ to 1 pound each), peeled and cut lengthwise into slices ½ inch thick

Coarse sea salt

6 tablespoons extra-virgin olive oil

½ cup basil leaves

½ cup crumbled sheep or goat's milk feta cheese

8 sun-dried tomato halves packed in oil, drained and coarsely chopped

12 pitted kalamata olives, chopped

½ cup shredded Pecorino Romano cheese

Sprinkle the eggplant slices lightly with salt on both sides and let drain in a colander for 30 to 60 minutes. Rinse under cold running water and dry well, pressing to remove as much moisture as possible.

Preheat the broiler. Brush the eggplant slices on both sides with 3 tablespoons of the oil and set on a baking sheet. Broil 3 to 4 inches from the heat, turning once, until lightly browned, 3 to 4 minutes on each side.

In a mini food processor, puree the basil with the remaining 3 tablespoons oil, or finely chop the basil and stir into the oil. Transfer to a small bowl and toss the basil oil with the feta, sun-dried tomatoes, and olives. Spread over the eggplant slices, dividing evenly. Sprinkle the Romano cheese on top.

Return to the broiler and broil briefly until the feta is hot and the cheese on top has melted and is just beginning to brown at the edges, about 1 minute.

Roasted Cauliflower and Radicchio in Anchovy-Garlic Sauce

4 SERVINGS | 4 POINTS EACH

Roasting vegetables is very popular lately, and with good reason. It's easy and develops wonderful flavors that turn formerly shunned vegetables, such as cauliflower and brussels sprouts, into newfound culinary superstars.

½ large head cauliflower, separated into florets (5 to 6 cups)

½ head radicchio, coarsely shredded (about 2 cups)

½ teaspoon sea salt

⅛ teaspoon freshly ground pepper

4 tablespoons extra-virgin olive oil

1 clove garlic, minced

6 flat anchovy fillets (about ¾ ounce), chopped

½ teaspoon minced fresh rosemary or crumbled dried

¼ teaspoon crushed hot red pepper

Preheat the oven to 375°F. In a shallow roasting pan or gratin dish, toss the cauliflower and radicchio with the salt, freshly ground pepper, and 2 tablespoons of the olive oil. Pour in ¼ cup of water and roast for 20 to 25 minutes, or until the cauliflower is tender and lightly browned in spots.

In a small saucepan, cook the garlic and anchovies in the remaining 2 tablespoons olive oil over medium heat until the garlic softens and the anchovies melt into the oil, 2 to 3 minutes. Add the rosemary and hot red pepper.

Pour the sauce over the vegetables, scraping all the oil from the pan. Toss briefly to coat and serve.

Eggplant Stuffed with Mozzarella and Prosciutto in Basil Tomato Sauce

8 SERVINGS AS A FIRST COURSE, 4 AS A MAIN DISH | 9 OR 18 POINTS EACH

This classic dish is based on the Eggplant Involtini in *The Tuscan Sun Cookbook* by Frances and Edward Mayes. If you'd prefer to enjoy it as a main course, serve two eggplant rolls per person and offer steamed broccoli and a small portion of pasta on the side.

Extra-virgin olive oil, for brushing

Basil Tomato Sauce (recipe follows)

1 large eggplant

1½ teaspoons dried oregano

Salt and freshly ground pepper

8 thin slices prosciutto

8 thin slices mozzarella cheese

⅓ cup grated Parmigiano-Reggiano cheese

Preheat the oven to 400°F. Line a large baking sheet with parchment and brush the parchment with oil.

Make the Basil Tomato Sauce. While the sauce is simmering, cut the eggplant into 8 slices about ⅜ inch thick. (Take your time cutting the eggplant so the slices are as even as possible.) Brush both sides of the slices with olive oil and arrange in a single layer on the baking sheet. Sprinkle the oregano over the eggplant and season lightly with salt and pepper. Bake the eggplant for 5 minutes. Carefully turn over and bake for 5 minutes longer, until the slices are tender but not mushy. Remove from the oven and let cool. Decrease the oven temperature to 350°F.

When the eggplant slices are cool enough to handle, place a slice of prosciutto and a slice of mozzarella on each. Starting at the smaller end, roll up and secure with a wooden toothpick or two.

Spread about ¾ cup of the tomato sauce over the bottom of a 9 by 12-inch baking dish. Arrange the eggplant rolls seam side down in the dish. Spoon more tomato sauce over each roll and sprinkle the Parmigiano-Reggiano over the top. Bake until the mozzarella is melted and the rolls are heated through, 15 to 20 minutes.

Basil Tomato Sauce

MAKES ABOUT 2½ CUPS; 8 SERVINGS | 1 POINT EACH

This quick-cooking tomato sauce uses a mixture of fresh and canned tomatoes for maximum flavor and texture.

4 Roma tomatoes	½ onion, finely chopped	1 tablespoon tomato paste
1 (28-ounce) can Italian peeled tomatoes	3 tablespoons extra-virgin olive oil	½ teaspoon sugar
½ cup lightly packed fresh basil leaves	4 cloves garlic, minced	Salt and freshly ground pepper
	¼ teaspoon crushed hot red pepper	

To peel the tomatoes, drop them into a small pot of boiling water for about 30 seconds. Rinse under cold running water; the skins should just slip off. Cut the tomatoes into ¼-inch dice. Set aside with any juices that exude.

Drain the canned tomatoes, reserving the juices. Put the tomatoes in a blender with ⅔ cup of the juices and the basil leaves. Pulse until coarsely chopped.

In a deep pot, cook the onion in the olive oil over medium-high heat, stirring often, until soft and golden, about 5 minutes. Add the garlic and hot red pepper and cook for 1 minute longer. Add the tomato paste and sugar and cook, stirring, until the paste darkens, about 2 minutes.

Pour the pureed tomatoes and the diced fresh tomatoes with their juices into the pot and stir to mix well. Bring to a boil, decrease the heat, and simmer for 10 to 15 minutes. Season with salt and pepper to taste.

Swiss Chard and Ricotta Torta

MAKES 1 (9-INCH) TART; 6 SERVINGS | 14 POINTS EACH

A crispy phyllo crust encases this quiche-like pie brimming with gutsy Italian flavors. Look for boxes of phyllo dough in the frozen foods section of large supermarkets. Once thawed, use only as many sheets as you need for the recipe; immediately return the rest to the freezer for another use. And don't worry if any of the sheets tear as you're working. This dough is very forgiving, so just patch the sheet back together and keep working.

2 tablespoons extra-virgin olive oil

1 onion, chopped

1 red bell pepper, seeded and cut into ½-inch dice

2 cloves garlic, minced

1 bunch green Swiss chard (about 8 ounces leaves and stems), trimmed and chopped

Salt

¼ teaspoon crushed hot red pepper

1 (15-ounce) container whole-milk ricotta cheese

3 eggs, lightly beaten

¼ cup freshly grated Parmesan cheese

2 tablespoons heavy cream

8 (17 by 12-inch) sheets phyllo dough (4 to 5 ounces), thawed as package directs

Preheat the oven to 350°F. Spray the bottom and sides of a 9-inch deep-dish pie plate with nonstick cooking spray.

In a large skillet, heat the oil over medium heat. Add the onion, bell pepper, and garlic and cook, stirring occasionally, until soft, 3 to 5 minutes. Add the chard, a handful or two at a time, stirring and letting the leaves wilt before adding more. When all of the chard has been added, season to taste with salt and stir in the hot red pepper. Decrease the heat to low. Cover the pan and cook until the chard is barely tender, about 5 minutes. Remove the pan from the heat, uncover, and let cool to room temperature.

In a large bowl, mix together the ricotta, eggs, Parmesan, cream, and ½ teaspoon salt. Scrape the chard mixture into the bowl. Stir until well blended.

Unfold the phyllo. Stack 8 sheets on a clean work surface and cover with plastic wrap. (Refrigerate or freeze the remaining phyllo sheets for another use.) Working quickly, place 1 sheet of phyllo in the center of the prepared pie plate. Use your fingers to ease the dough into the plate, pressing the dough against the bottom and sides for a snug fit and letting the corners of the phyllo sheet drape over the edge. Spray the dough all over with the cooking spray. Turn the dish about a quarter-turn and add a second sheet of phyllo, once again pressing it into the dish to form a pastry shell. Continue turning the pie plate a quarter-turn and layering and spraying the sheets with oil, making sure that eventually there is an overhang of phyllo all around the outside edge of the dish.

Scrape the chard mixture into the pastry shell, spreading into an even layer. Fold and crimp the overhanging dough to form a rustic edge. (Don't aim for perfection here; it will look great once baked.) Spray the folded edge with cooking spray. Bake until the pastry is golden and the filling is set and slightly puffy, about 40 minutes. If the pastry begins to brown too quickly, cover loosely with foil. Let the torta stand for at least 15 minutes before cutting into wedges. Serve warm or at room temperature.

Kale Salad with Sweet Potato "Croutons"

5 SERVINGS | 8 POINTS EACH

Unlike most salad greens, kale benefits from being dressed in advance, letting the oil and vinegar tenderize the leaves. Every bite here celebrates the arrival of fall, with harmonious elements like pumpkin and cranberry dotted with roasted sweet potatoes and bits of creamy goat cheese.

12 ounces red-skinned sweet potatoes (yams), peeled and cut into 1-inch chunks

1 small red onion, cut into ½-inch-thick slices

4 tablespoons extra-virgin olive oil

Salt and freshly ground pepper

1 tablespoon sherry wine vinegar

1 small clove garlic, crushed through a press

8 cups (lightly packed) baby kale (about 12 ounces)

3 tablespoons hulled green pumpkin seeds (pepitas)

½ cup crumbled soft goat cheese (about 2 ounces)

2 tablespoons dried cranberries

Preheat the oven to 425°F. On a large baking sheet, combine the sweet potatoes and red onion. Drizzle with 1 tablespoon of the oil and season with salt and pepper to taste. Spread out the vegetables in an even layer and bake, stirring once or twice and breaking the onion slices into rings, until the sweet potatoes are nicely browned at the edges and tender when pierced with the tip of a sharp knife, about 25 minutes. Let cool to room temperature.

Meanwhile, in a large bowl, combine the vinegar, garlic, ¼ teaspoon salt, and a generous grinding of pepper. Whisk in the remaining 3 tablespoons olive oil. Add the kale and toss to coat evenly with the dressing. (If made in advance, cover and let stand at room temperature for up to 2 hours, or refrigerate for up to 6 hours.)

In a dry heavy skillet, toast the pumpkin seeds over medium heat, stirring frequently, until puffed and golden, 3 to 4 minutes. Let cool.

To serve, scrape the onion and sweet potato mixture into the kale along with any cooking juices that may have accumulated on the baking sheet. Add the pumpkin seeds, goat cheese, and dried cranberries. Toss gently to mix.

Roasted Winter Vegetables

6 SERVINGS | 5 POINTS EACH

Buy a rotisserie chicken, throw a pan of these wonderful vegetables into the oven, and with little effort, you have an entire dinner ready and waiting for you. Other vegetables that could be included in your pan are parsnips, rutabaga, fresh fennel, and celery root (celeriac).

12 ounces Yukon gold potatoes (2 or 3)

3 carrots, peeled

1 onion, cut into 8 to 10 wedges

16 to 20 brussels sprouts, trimmed and halved

2 tablespoons extra-virgin olive oil

¼ teaspoon crushed hot red pepper

Coarse sea salt and freshly ground pepper

⅓ cup chicken broth

6 sprigs fresh rosemary

4 to 6 whole cloves garlic

Preheat the oven to 400°F. Cut the potatoes and carrots into 1- to 1½-inch chunks.

In a large roasting pan, combine the potatoes, carrots, onion, and brussels sprouts. Toss to mix. Drizzle on the olive oil and sprinkle on the hot red pepper. Season generously with salt and freshly ground pepper. Add the broth. Tuck the rosemary and garlic into the vegetables, distributing them around the pan.

Roast, stirring once or twice, until the vegetables are tender and lightly browned, 25 to 35 minutes.

Lemony Stir-Fried Brussels Sprouts

4 SERVINGS | 3 POINTS EACH

Roasted brussels sprouts are all the rage. True, they're easy, but they do take a lot of time. This marvelous dish, which leaves the sprouts bright green and just slightly crisp, requires a little slicing, but then it's on the table in less than 10 minutes.

12 ounces fresh brussels sprouts

½ onion, thinly sliced

1 shallot, thinly sliced

3 tablespoons extra-virgin olive oil

Sea salt

3 tablespoons freshly squeezed lemon juice

Trim the stems off the brussels sprouts. Cut each into thin slices.

In a wok or large cast-iron skillet, cook the onion and shallot in the oil over high heat, stirring occasionally, until the onion is soft and just beginning to color, about 3 minutes.

Add the sprouts and season with ½ teaspoon of salt. Continue to cook, tossing, for 2 minutes. Pour ½ cup of water into the wok, cover, and decrease the heat to medium. Cook for 3 to 5 minutes, or until the sprouts are just tender but still bright green.

Remove from the heat. Season with the lemon juice and additional salt to taste.

Savory Lentils with Mushrooms and Dill

4 SERVINGS | 5 POINTS EACH

While this preparation is included as an essential component for our Salmon-Stuffed Cabbage (page 169), it makes a fabulous side dish for almost any poultry or meat. At room temperature, it could be your protein component of a nice salad. Sprinkled with a little feta or goat cheese, it makes an excellent vegetarian main course.

¾ cup chopped onion

2 tablespoons extra-virgin olive oil

¾ cup chopped celery

¾ cup finely diced carrot

½ cup finely diced parsnip

¼ teaspoon dried thyme

Sea salt and freshly ground pepper

½ cup small French green lentils

1 cup chicken broth

1 cup water

1½ ounces dried mushrooms, chopped or crumbled (about 3 tablespoons)

1 small bay leaf

1 tablespoon white wine vinegar

⅓ cup coarsely chopped fresh dill

Sauté the onion in the olive oil over medium-high heat until softened and golden, about 5 minutes. Add the celery, carrot, and parsnip. Continue to cook until the vegetables are softened, 7 to 10 minutes. Season with the thyme, salt, and pepper.

Add the lentils and pour in the broth and water. Add the dried mushrooms and tuck the bay leaf into the mixture. Bring to a boil, decrease the heat to a simmer, and cook, partially covered, for 25 minutes.

Stir in the vinegar. Remove from the heat and let stand, covered, until most of the liquid is absorbed and the lentils are tender but still slightly resistant to the bite, about 10 minutes. Season with additional salt and pepper to taste. Remove the bay leaf. Stir in the dill shortly before serving.

rovençal Vegetable Salad with Chickpeas and Basil

5 SERVINGS | 3 POINTS EACH

Here's a light, flavorful salad that can serve as a side dish or, topped with a bit of feta cheese and spooned on top of greens, as a main course salad. The vegetables will taste more flavorful if they marinate in the dressing for a while.

3 ounces green beans, preferably thin *haricots verts*, trimmed and cut into ¾-inch pieces

1 large carrot, peeled and cut into ½-inch dice

1 cup small cauliflower florets

1 zucchini, cut into ¾-inch dice

1 small shallot, minced

1 tablespoon red wine vinegar

2 teaspoons freshly squeezed lemon juice

Sea salt and freshly ground pepper

½ teaspoon Dijon mustard

3 tablespoons extra-virgin olive oil

½ red bell pepper, seeded and cut into ½-inch dice

½ cup canned chickpeas

3 tablespoons chopped fresh basil or parsley

In a steamer pot over boiling water, steam the green beans for 4 minutes, or until just tender; rinse briefly under cold running water to cool and transfer to a colander to drain. In the same pot, steam the carrot and cauliflower until just tender, about 3 minutes; rinse to cool and transfer to the colander. Lastly, steam the zucchini until barely tender, 2 to 3 minutes; rinse and drain well.

Put the shallot in a bowl. Pour the vinegar and lemon juice over the shallot and season with ¼ teaspoon each of salt and pepper. Whisk in the mustard, then slowly whisk in the olive oil.

Add the steamed vegetables to the dressing. Add the bell pepper, chickpeas, and half the basil to the salad and toss to mix. Season with additional salt and pepper to taste. Sprinkle the remaining basil on top just before serving.

Spicy Black Bean Chili

4 SERVINGS | 3 POINTS EACH

Here's an easily assembled vegetarian chili sure to warm your soul. It's delicious as is, and even better when tamed with a sprinkling of shredded cheese or a dollop of sour cream on top. For complete protein, serve over a small portion of brown rice. Chopped scallions or cilantro make colorful garnishes on the side.

1 tablespoon extra-virgin olive oil	1 clove garlic, finely chopped	½ teaspoon dried oregano
2 zucchini, chopped	1 teaspoon chipotle chile powder	1 (15-ounce) can black beans, rinsed well and drained
2 celery ribs, chopped	½ teaspoon salt	
1 onion, chopped	½ teaspoon ground cumin	1 (10-ounce) can diced tomatoes with green chiles
1 red or green bell pepper, seeded and chopped		

In a large saucepan, warm the oil over medium heat. Add the zucchini, celery, onion, bell pepper, garlic, chipotle chile powder, salt, cumin, and oregano. Cook, stirring occasionally, until the vegetables are softened but not browned, about 10 minutes.

Add the black beans; use a wooden spoon to mash about half of them against the sides of the pan. Stir in the tomatoes with chiles and their juices and ½ cup of water. Bring to a boil, decrease the heat to low, and cook, stirring occasionally, until the vegetables are tender and the chili has thickened slightly, 10 to 15 minutes. Serve at once, or refrigerate or freeze.

Zucchini Succotash

6 SERVINGS | 3 POINTS EACH

This high-fiber vegetable mélange is colorful and tasty, perfect for pairing with grilled chicken or fish. Use fresh corn in season, vacuum-packed in winter.

1 onion, chopped	1 teaspoon cumin seeds, crushed	¾ cup corn kernels
2 tablespoons extra-virgin olive oil	¼ to ½ teaspoon crushed hot red pepper, to taste	½ teaspoon ground cumin
½ green bell pepper, seeded and diced		½ teaspoon dried oregano
½ red bell pepper, seeded and diced	1 (15-ounce) can diced tomatoes	¼ cup chicken broth, vegetable stock, or water
3 cloves garlic, finely chopped	3 zucchini (about 12 ounces total), sliced or diced	Sea salt and freshly ground pepper

In a large skillet, sauté the onion in the olive oil over medium-high heat until soft and golden, 5 to 7 minutes. Add the bell peppers, garlic, cumin seeds, and hot red pepper. Cook for 3 minutes longer.

Add the tomatoes and simmer for 10 minutes. Add the zucchini, corn, ground cumin, and oregano. Pour in the broth, cover, and bring to a boil. Decrease the heat and simmer, partially covered, until the zucchini are just tender, about 5 minutes longer. Season with salt and pepper to taste

WHOLE GRAINS AND PASTA

A number of popular diets, most notably the Paleo diet, shun all grains. The science behind the claims that cave dwellers and other prehistoric people were healthier because they did not eat cultivated grains has been refuted over and over. First of all, early humans did eat plant carbohydrates; and second, their remains have shown signs of heart disease, arthritis, and cancer. Also, most chronic diseases tend to arise after the age of forty, and these early humans, with no sanitary systems or electricity, chasing mastodons for dinner, could not have lived very long. Yet many people cling to the belief that giving up grains will improve their digestion.

The truth is, whole grains in appropriate amounts are associated with better health and better glycemic control. They provide valuable nutrients—especially B vitamins, zinc, magnesium, and vital fibers—and are high in the essential amino acid methionine, which, when combined with another essential amino acid, lysine (found in large quantities in beans), makes carnitine, an important chemical for burning fats and cleaning up the toxins produced by that combustion.

Dilled Barley Salad with Corn and Edamame

4 SERVINGS AS A MAIN, 8 SERVINGS AS A SIDE | 8 OR 4 POINTS EACH

This dish combines fabulous texture and valuable protein in a tasty vegetarian package. Enjoy as a main dish or an interesting side. Because it's dressed simply with oil and vinegar, it makes a great choice for a tailgate or picnic.

1 cup pearled barley	1 cup frozen edamame (shelled soybeans)	¼ cup minced red onion
1¾ cups chicken or vegetable broth	3 tablespoons sherry or wine vinegar	¼ cup chopped fresh dill
1 cup fresh or frozen corn kernels	3 tablespoons extra-virgin olive oil	Salt and freshly ground pepper

In a small saucepan over medium heat, cook the barley in the broth and ¾ cup of water until the barley is tender but remains pleasingly chewy, 20 to 25 minutes.

Meanwhile, steam the corn until just tender, 2 to 3 minutes. Remove and rinse under cold running water. Steam the frozen edamame until just hot and tender but not mushy, 2 to 3 minutes. Drain and rinse to stop the cooking; drain well.

In a serving bowl, toss the barley with the vinegar, olive oil, red onion, and 3 tablespoons of the dill. Season with salt and pepper to taste.

Add the corn and edamame and fold gently to mix. Sprinkle the remaining 1 tablespoon of dill on top. Serve warm or at room temperature.

Portobello Mushrooms Stuffed with Eggplant, Barley, and Feta Cheese

4 SERVINGS | 5 POINTS EACH

Here's a marvelous vegetarian main course. Serve hot from the oven along with a mixed green salad loaded with thinly sliced cucumber, radishes, and Belgian endive and dressed in a lemony vinaigrette.

¼ cup pearled barley

4 portobello mushrooms (about 4 inches across)

4 teaspoons soy sauce

4 teaspoons plus 2 tablespoons extra-virgin olive oil

2½ tablespoons pine nuts (pignoli)

4 small, narrow Asian eggplants (about 1 pound total), chopped

1 onion, chopped

1 red or yellow bell pepper, seeded and cut into ½-inch squares

2 celery ribs, chopped

2 cloves garlic, finely chopped

Salt and freshly ground pepper

2 oil-packed sun-dried tomato halves, finely chopped (about 2 tablespoons)

6 tablespoons crumbled feta cheese (about 2 ounces)

2 teaspoons chopped flat-leaf parsley

Preheat the oven to 400°F. Line a baking sheet with parchment.

In a small saucepan of salted water, cook the barley until tender but not mushy, 20 to 25 minutes. Drain in a fine sieve.

Meanwhile, wipe the mushroom caps clean with a damp paper towel. If there are stems, remove them, trim off the ends, and chop; set aside. Using a melon baller or a spoon, scrape out and discard the dark gills inside the mushroom cap.

In a small bowl, mix together the soy sauce and 4 teaspoons of the oil. Brush over both sides of the mushroom caps. Place the caps stem side down on the prepared baking sheet and bake until barely browned at the edges, 4 to 5 minutes. Set aside to cool slightly. Leave the oven on.

In a large dry skillet, toast the pine nuts over low heat, stirring and shaking the pan constantly, until lightly browned, 2 to 3 minutes. Remove the pine nuts from the skillet and set aside.

continued

ortobello Mushrooms, continued

In the same skillet, heat the remaining 2 tablespoons oil over medium heat. Add the chopped mushroom stems (if any) and the eggplant, onion, bell pepper, celery, and garlic. Season with ½ teaspoon of salt and a generous grinding of pepper. Cook, stirring occasionally, until the eggplant is very tender, 7 to 9 minutes. Remove from the heat and stir in the barley, toasted pine nuts, and sun-dried tomatoes. Season with additional salt and pepper to taste.

Arrange the mushrooms, stem sides up, in a small baking pan. Fill the cavities with the eggplant-barley mixture, mounding slightly. Top each with 1½ tablespoons of the crumbled feta cheese. Return the mushrooms to the hot oven and bake until the filling is heated through and the cheese is soft, 7 to 10 minutes. Sprinkle with the parsley and serve at once.

Wheat Berry Salad

6 SERVINGS | 4 POINTS EACH

Wheat berries may take a bit of time to cook, but it's an easy task that's well worth the great payoff in texture and fiber that comes in at a mere 4 points per serving.

⅔ cup wheat berries

¼ cup extra-virgin olive oil

1 red onion, chopped

1 clove garlic, finely chopped

1 tablespoon balsamic vinegar

1 yellow or red bell pepper, seeded and cut into ½-inch dice

2 celery ribs, chopped

1 small cucumber, peeled if desired, seeded, and cut into ½-inch dice

Salt and freshly ground pepper

1½ cups cherry or grape tomatoes cut into halves or quarters (about 8 ounces)

In a saucepan, bring about 4 cups of salted water to a boil over medium-high heat. Stir in the wheat berries and return to a boil. Decrease the heat to low and cook, uncovered, until tender but still slightly chewy, about 45 minutes. Drain well.

In a skillet, heat 1 tablespoon of the oil over medium heat. Add the onion and garlic and cook, stirring occasionally, until the onion is softened but not browned, 3 to 5 minutes. Remove from the heat and stir in the vinegar and the remaining 3 tablespoons of oil.

In a large bowl, mix together the warm wheat berries, the onion mixture, bell pepper, celery, cucumber, ½ teaspoon of salt, and pepper to taste. Add the cherry tomatoes and toss gently to mix. Cover and let stand for 30 minutes at room temperature to blend flavors. (If made in advance, the salad can be refrigerated for up to 8 hours and returned to cool room temperature.) Before serving, stir gently and taste, adding more salt or pepper if needed.

Asparagus Risotto

6 SERVINGS | 8 POINTS EACH

Keep in mind that this counts as one of your refined carbohydrates for the week, so it should be served only as a special treat. It's going to cost you dearly on your budget, but once in a while you'll decide it's worth it.

1 large bunch asparagus (about 1¼ pounds)

1 large shallot, finely chopped

2 tablespoons extra-virgin olive oil

1 cup Arborio rice

About 5 cups hot vegetable or chicken broth

¼ teaspoon freshly grated nutmeg

Dash of cayenne pepper

2 tablespoons unsalted butter

6 tablespoons grated Parmigiano-Reggiano cheese

Sea salt and freshly ground pepper

Trim off the tough stem ends from the asparagus and thinly slice the spears crosswise, leaving about 1 inch of the tips intact. Set the tips aside separately.

In a heavy saucepan or flameproof casserole, cook the shallot in the olive oil over medium heat, stirring once or twice, until softened, about 2 minutes. Add the rice and cook, stirring often, for 2 minutes longer.

Pour in ½ cup of the hot broth. Add the nutmeg and cayenne. Cook, stirring, until most of the liquid evaporates. Add the sliced asparagus stalks and ¾ cup broth and continue to cook, stirring occasionally, until most of the liquid is absorbed. Repeat, adding more broth as needed, until the rice has cooked for 10 minutes.

Add the asparagus tips and more broth and continue to cook until the rice is tender but still firm and the "sauce" around it is thick and creamy, about 8 minutes longer.

Stir in the butter and cheese. Season lightly with salt and generously with freshly ground pepper. Serve immediately.

Asian Quinoa with Spinach and Mushrooms

4 SERVINGS | 4 POINTS EACH

While quinoa is a grain—by definition high in starch—it is also high in fiber and protein. Plus, it's paired here with vegetables, so you can enjoy either a nice ¾-cup serving as a side dish or a cup if you're having it as a vegetarian main dish.

⅔ cup quinoa, preferably red	1 clove garlic, minced	2 teaspoons soy sauce
8 ounces white button mushrooms, quartered	6 ounces prewashed baby spinach or baby kale	1 teaspoon rice vinegar
2 tablespoons extra-virgin olive oil		1 teaspoon toasted sesame oil

If the quinoa is not prerinsed, put it in a bowl and pour 2 cups of hot water over it. Swish it around and drain into a fine sieve; repeat.

Put the quinoa in a saucepan. Add 1⅓ cups of water, bring to a boil, and decrease the heat to low. Cover and simmer for 10 minutes.

Meanwhile, in a skillet, sauté the mushrooms in the olive oil over medium-high heat until they give up their juices and start to brown, 3 to 5 minutes. Add the garlic and sauté for 30 seconds longer. Scrape the mushrooms and garlic into the quinoa and continue cooking until the quinoa is tender and the little tails uncurl, 5 to 10 minutes.

Stir in the spinach, cover, and remove from the heat. Let stand for 3 minutes. Stir in the soy sauce, vinegar, and sesame oil. Serve hot or at room temperature.

Quinoa with Cranberries and Kale

6 SERVINGS | 6 POINTS EACH

This is a lovely salad that could make a complete lunch with perhaps a small wedge of feta cheese, followed by a piece of fruit for dessert. It's also a fine side dish for chicken, turkey, or fish.

¾ cup quinoa	2 scallions, minced	2 teaspoons soy sauce
1½ cups chicken or vegetable broth	4 ounces baby kale, well rinsed and dried	Salt and freshly ground pepper
½ cup dried cranberries or currants	2 teaspoons toasted sesame oil	

If the quinoa is not prerinsed, put it in a bowl and pour 2 cups of hot water over it. Swish it around and drain into a fine sieve; repeat.

In a small saucepan, bring the broth to a boil. Add the quinoa, decrease the heat to low, cover, and cook until the little tails partially uncurl and the grain is just tender, 12 to 15 minutes.

Remove from the heat. Stir in the cranberries, scallions, and baby kale. Let stand, covered, for about 2 minutes.

Transfer the quinoa mixture to a serving bowl. Add the sesame oil and soy sauce and toss to coat. Season, if needed, with salt and pepper to taste.

Parmesan Polenta

6 SERVINGS | 8 POINTS EACH

If you're from the South, you'll know this as grits. Cornmeal is not low in carbohydrate for sure, but it is a whole grain with valuable antioxidants. In the context of a healthy diet, it is a fine choice in appropriate portions, especially when paired, as it is here, with protein and some fat. Serve plain as an accompaniment, or turn into "croutons" (see recipe below) to use as a base for poached eggs, a tomato-based sauce, stewed greens, or a mushroom ragout.

3½ to 4 cups chicken or vegetable stock or water	¾ cup yellow cornmeal 1 teaspoon salt Dash of cayenne pepper	2 tablespoon unsalted butter ½ cup grated Parmesan cheese

Pour 2 cups of the stock into a saucepan and bring to a boil over medium-high heat. In a bowl, stir the cornmeal into 1½ cups of cold stock. Gradually add this cornmeal slurry to the boiling hot stock in a thin stream, stirring it in constantly so no lumps form.

Decrease the heat to medium and cook, stirring, until the cornmeal thickens and begins to pull away from the sides of the pan, 20 to 25 minutes. Add more stock if needed. If the thick bubbling mixture starts splattering, decrease the heat slightly.

When the polenta is tender, season with the salt and cayenne. Add the butter and stir until melted. Remove from the heat and stir in the cheese. Serve at once.

POLENTA CROUTONS: Spread out the hot cooked polenta on a platter or in a baking pan to an even ½ inch. Let stand until set, 10 to 15 minutes. The firm polenta can be covered and refrigerated for several hours or overnight.

Cut the firm polenta into 2½- to 3-inch rounds or squares. Brush with olive oil and broil until hot and browned on top, or sauté in a lightly oiled cast-iron pan, turning once, until golden brown on both sides.

Black Bean and Veggie Burgers
with Bulgur and Oats

MAKES 10 (3-INCH) PATTIES; 5 SERVINGS | 8 POINTS EACH

This includes lots of ingredients to get the texture just right, but it's not a lot of work. The burger mixture needs to be chilled so it sets up before cooking, so allow time for refrigeration. Serve these as you would any other burger—perhaps with a slather of Dijon mustard, plenty of lettuce, sliced tomato, and onion, along with a juicy dill pickle on the side. Individually wrap any leftover cooked burgers and keep them in your freezer.

¾ cup bulgur

1 (15-ounce) can black beans, rinsed well and drained

½ cup walnut halves and pieces, finely chopped

¼ cup rolled oats (old-fashioned or quick-cooking oatmeal)

2 tablespoons soy sauce

1 tablespoon tomato paste

3 tablespoons extra-virgin olive oil

8 ounces mushrooms, finely chopped

2 small zucchini, finely chopped

1 carrot, finely chopped

½ onion, finely chopped

2 cloves garlic, minced

1 teaspoon salt

⅛ teaspoon cayenne pepper

1 egg, lightly beaten

In a bowl, combine the bulgur with enough hot water to cover by 1 inch. Let stand until softened, 10 to 15 minutes. Drain well in a fine sieve.

In a large bowl, combine the bulgur, beans, walnuts, oats, soy sauce, and tomato paste. Mash with a fork until blended but not completely smooth.

In a large sauté pan or skillet, heat 2 tablespoons of the olive oil over medium-high heat. Add the mushrooms, zucchini, carrot, onion, and garlic. Season with the salt and cayenne. Cook, stirring occasionally and adjusting the heat as needed to prevent burning, until the vegetables are tender, 8 to 10 minutes. Scrape the vegetables into the bean mixture and let cool for 5 minutes. Stir to combine, then stir in the egg and mix until well blended.

Spray a baking sheet with nonstick cooking spray. Using a large ice cream scoop or a ½-cup measure, scoop mounds of the mixture onto the baking sheet. Use a spatula to gently pat down the top of each mound, forming a 3-inch patty about ½ inch thick. Cover with plastic wrap and refrigerate until firm, at least 4 hours or overnight.

In a large nonstick skillet, heat the remaining 1 tablespoon of oil over medium heat. Working in batches, add the patties to the skillet without crowding. Cook, turning once or twice, until heated through and nicely browned all over, 10 to 12 minutes total. Repeat with the remaining patties, adding more oil to the pan if needed.

Pasta Puttenesca

6 SERVINGS | 15 POINTS EACH

Simple and vegetarian, this dish can be made into more of a substantial first course by adding a drained can of tuna at the end or—better yet—chunks of grilled fresh tuna. There are several brands of high-fiber pastas, which are bulked up with extra fiber called inulin that cannot be digested, so it dilutes the carbohydrate load. Make sure the pasta is cooked al dente, and pass cheese on the side if you like.

3 cloves garlic, thinly sliced

¼ cup extra-virgin olive oil

3 tablespoons tiny (nonpareil) capers

6 anchovy fillets, chopped

¼ to ½ teaspoon crushed hot red pepper, to taste

1 (28-ounce) can chopped tomatoes with their juices

12 pitted kalamata olives, slivered or sliced

Salt and freshly ground pepper

12 ounces thin high-fiber spaghetti, such as Dreamfields

⅓ cup coarsely chopped parsley

In a large skillet or flameproof casserole, cook the garlic in the olive oil over medium heat until softened and fragrant, about 2 minutes. Add the capers, anchovies, and hot red pepper, and cook, stirring, until the anchovies dissolve, about 1 minute.

Add the tomatoes and olives. Raise the heat to high and bring to a boil. Decrease to a simmer and cook for 10 to 15 minutes to reduce slightly. Season with salt and pepper to taste.

Meanwhile, bring a large pot of salted water to a boil. Add the pasta and cook until it is just tender but still slightly resistant to the bite, 9 to 11 minutes; test often. Immediately drain the pasta into a large colander.

Stir ¼ cup of the parsley into the sauce. Add the pasta and toss with tongs. Simmer for 2 minutes. Transfer to a large serving bowl and sprinkle the remaining 4 teaspoons of parsley on top.

Tabbouleh

6 SERVINGS | 6 POINTS EACH

Almost more greens than grains, this wonderful Middle Eastern salad is best served at room temperature or only slightly chilled.

---

1 cup bulgur or medium cracked wheat

7 tablespoons extra-virgin olive oil

3 to 4 tablespoons freshly squeezed lemon juice

Coarse (kosher) salt and freshly ground pepper

1 cup coarsely chopped fresh flat-leaf parsley

½ cup chopped fresh mint

⅓ cup minced scallions (white and green parts) or ¼ cup minced red onion

3 or 4 ripe plum tomatoes, finely diced

Rinse the bulgur in a strainer under cold running water. Transfer to a bowl, cover with cold water, and let stand until softened but still firm, about 45 minutes. Drain well. Squeeze out as much excess water as possible.

In a bowl, toss the bulgur with 6 tablespoons of the olive oil, 3 tablespoons of the lemon juice, 1 teaspoon of salt, and ¼ teaspoon of pepper.

Add the parsley, mint, scallions, and tomatoes. Toss well to mix. Season with additional salt, pepper, and lemon juice to taste. Shortly before serving, drizzle the remaining 1 tablespoon of olive oil over the top.

SWEET TREATS

Just because you have elevated blood sugar or have received a diagnosis of type 2 diabetes doesn't mean you're *never* going to eat anything sweet again. Choose your desserts wisely so that, ideally, you are getting some good nutrition from them. Take a good look at the number of servings, and do practice strict portion control. Savor every bite. Eat sugar only after a full meal, so that you don't get an insulin rush from all that sugar on an empty stomach. And do make sure your sweet treat is just that: a once-a-week occurrence that you enjoy because it is so special. Other days of the week, satisfy your craving with fruit and cheese, fruit and nuts, a fruit ice pop, or a small square of dark chocolate.

Baked Apples with Walnuts and Maple Syrup

4 SERVINGS | 12 POINTS EACH

There are so many interesting varieties of apples available now. Choose one that is flavorful, with enough tartness to balance the sweeteners and firm enough to stand up to baking without falling apart. Cortlands and Rome Beauties are traditional baking apples; Granny Smiths also work well. Serve these on their own or topped with a dollop of vanilla yogurt.

4 baking apples (4 to 6 ounces each)	¼ cup dried currants	2 tablespoons maple syrup
⅓ cup chopped walnuts	1 teaspoon ground cinnamon	4 teaspoons unsalted butter

Preheat the oven to 375°F. Core the apples, leaving about ½ inch intact at the bottom. Peel off about one-third of the skin from the top half. Using a grapefruit knife, carve out some of the apple, leaving about a ¾-inch shell. Chop the apple you've taken out.

In a small bowl, toss the chopped apple with the walnuts, currants, and cinnamon. Fill the apples with this mixture, dividing evenly. Drizzle 1½ teaspoons maple syrup into each apple. Top each with 1 teaspoon butter.

Arrange the apples in a small baking pan filled with ½ inch very hot water. Bake until the apples are tender but still hold their shape, 35 to 45 minutes, basting the apples with the pan juices once or twice. Serve warm, at room temperature, or chilled, with some of the pan juices drizzled on top.

Pecan Meringue Torte with Kiwi and Berries

There's no avoiding some sugar in a meringue, but this light dessert features fresh fruit and a touch of cream along with plenty of healthy pecans. Because nut meringue does not hold well, it's a good choice for a dinner party, which will ensure there are no leftovers to tempt you the next day.

---

3 large egg whites, at room temperature

⅛ teaspoon salt

⅛ teaspoon cream of tartar

⅓ cup granulated sugar

1 teaspoon vanilla extract

1 cup finely chopped pecans

½ cup heavy cream

2 tablespoons (1 ounce) cream cheese, softened

2 tablespoons confectioners' sugar

½ cup pureed strawberries or raspberries

1 pint strawberries, halved or sliced lengthwise

2 kiwis, peeled and sliced crosswise

½ cup blueberries

Preheat the oven to 300°F. Lightly butter an 8-inch pie pan and chill a bowl and beaters.

In a large bowl, whip the egg whites with the salt and cream of tartar until frothy. Gradually beat in the granulated sugar and continue whipping until the meringue forms very stiff peaks. Beat in ½ teaspoon of the vanilla. Fold in the chopped pecans. Spoon the nut meringue into the buttered pie pan and use a rubber or silicone spatula to smooth it up against the sides to form a shell, building up the edges as much as you can.

Bake for 35 to 40 minutes, until the shell is lightly browned. Set aside on a rack and let cool completely.

In the chilled bowl with the chilled beaters, whip the cream with the cream cheese and confectioners' sugar until stiff. Add the remaining ½ teaspoon vanilla and blend well. Beat in the pureed berries, then cover and refrigerate until ready to serve.

To assemble the tart, spread the vanilla whipped cream over the bottom of the nut meringue shell. Arrange the strawberries and kiwis decoratively around the rim of the shell and pile the blueberries in the center. Serve immediately.

Creamy Cannoli Cups

6 SERVINGS | 15 POINTS EACH

This recipe is a play on the classic Sicilian dessert, only with a much healthier twist. Instead of deep-fried pastry shells, the crunch comes from store-bought wonton wrappers, brushed lightly with oil and baked in a cupcake tin. With a few fresh raspberries on each plate, this makes a lovely, light dessert. Look for packages of wonton wrappers in the refrigerated section of Asian markets and in most well-stocked supermarkets. Extra wraps can be frozen for future use.

---

2 tablespoons coarsely chopped natural almonds (about 15 whole almonds)

6 (3¼-inch square) wonton wrappers

1½ teaspoons sunflower oil

1 (15-ounce) container whole-milk ricotta cheese

1 tablespoon brown rice syrup or honey

1 teaspoon finely grated orange zest

½ teaspoon vanilla extract

¼ teaspoon ground cinnamon

Dash of salt

2 tablespoons grated or finely chopped semisweet chocolate or semisweet mini morsels (mini chocolate chips)

Cocoa or espresso powder, for sprinkling (optional)

Preheat the oven to 350°F. Spread out the almonds in a small baking dish and toast, stirring once or twice, until lightly browned and fragrant, 5 to 7 minutes. Set aside. Do not turn off the oven.

Lay the wonton wrappers flat on a work surface and brush each with about ¼ teaspoon of the oil. Working 1 at a time, ease each wrapper, oiled side down, into a standard-size (2½-inch) muffin cup, pressing down to form a cup and pleating the sides as needed. When all 6 cups are formed, bake just until crisp and golden, 7 to 9 minutes. Let cool in the pan for 1 minute, then transfer to a rack to cool completely. (Cooled cups can be stored airtight at room temperature for up to 2 days.)

In a food processor, combine the ricotta, brown rice syrup, orange zest, vanilla, cinnamon, and salt. Process until the ricotta is smooth. Add the chocolate and process, pulsing the machine on and off 2 or 3 times, until incorporated. Scrape the mixture into a small bowl. (The filling can be refrigerated, covered, for up to 2 days.)

Just before serving, stir in the toasted almonds. Mound about ⅓ cup of filling into each wonton cup. Sprinkle with cocoa powder, if desired. Serve immediately.

Hazelnut Torte

Hazelnut flour, also called hazelnut meal or finely ground hazelnuts, is sold packaged and in bulk in some supermarkets. You can also grind your own flour in a food processor, using a couple of tablespoons of sugar from the recipe to prevent it from clumping. *Note:* This recipe contains a substantial amount of sugar, but portions are small, and the carbohydrate is buffered by the protein and fat in the eggs and nuts. Serve the cake plain or with a thin drizzle of melted bittersweet chocolate, or pass a bowl of Gingered Berry Compote (recipe opposite) on the side.

8 extra-large eggs, separated	1 teaspoon vanilla extract	½ teaspoon almond extract
¾ cup sugar	½ teaspoon orange extract	8 ounces hazelnut flour

Preheat the oven to 325°F. Butter a 10-inch springform pan. Line the bottom of the pan with parchment or waxed paper. Lightly butter the paper.

In a large bowl, beat the egg yolks lightly. Gradually beat in the sugar and continue beating until the mixture is light in color and falls from the beater in a slowly dissolving ribbon, 3 to 5 minutes. Beat in the vanilla, orange extract, and almond extract.

Beat the egg whites until stiff but not dry; watch carefully—overbeating will deflate the cake. Sprinkle about one-third of the ground nut flour over the egg yolk mixture. Scoop about one-third of the egg whites on top. Fold until partially blended. Repeat with half the remaining nut flour and egg whites. Then add the rest of the nut flour and egg whites and fold just until the mixture is blended and no streaks are visible.

Turn the batter into the prepared pan and bake in the upper third of the oven until the cake is puffed and browned and slightly springy to the touch, about 45 minutes. Let cool in the pan on a large rack for 5 minutes.

Run a dull knife around the rim of the pan to make sure the edges are loose. Remove the sides of the springform. Carefully invert to unmold the cake onto a plate. Gently peel off the paper. Invert back onto the rack and let cool.

Gingered Berry Compote

6 SERVINGS AS A DESSERT, 12 SERVINGS AS A SAUCE | 10 OR 5 POINTS EACH

Keep in mind, the sweeter the berries, the less sugar you will need to add. For a light dessert, stir 1 to 2 cups diced fresh fruit into the compote shortly before serving: peaches, nectarines, raspberries, and banana go especially well. As a sauce, spoon a few tablespoons over a simple cake or frozen yogurt.

2 pints (1 quart) flavorful ripe strawberries

1 cup blueberries

4 to 7 tablespoons demerara or turbinado sugar

¼ cup finely diced or chopped crystallized ginger

2 teaspoons balsamic vinegar

Rinse, hull, and quarter the strawberries. Place half in a small saucepan. Rinse and drain the blueberries; set them aside.

Add 4 tablespoons of the sugar and the ginger, vinegar, and ⅓ cup of water to the pan. Bring to a boil over medium heat. Boil, mashing lightly with a spoon to break up some of the berries. Decrease the heat and simmer, stirring occasionally, until the berries break down into a sauce, about 3 minutes.

Depending on the level of sweetness in the berries, add up to 3 more tablespoons of sugar to taste, 2 teaspoons at a time. Remove from the heat and add the remaining strawberries and the blueberries to the hot sauce. Let stand until cool. If not using shortly, cover and refrigerate until serving time. Serve chilled or at room temperature.

Grilled Peaches with Balsamic Glaze

Grilling fruit brings out its flavor, caramelizing the natural goodness for added depth. This recipe works really well for nectarines, too. You could serve these plain, with some farmstead cheese on the side, or present them as suggested here with a creamy topping.

---

4 ripe peaches

¼ cup balsamic vinegar

3 tablespoons dark brown sugar

¼ cup full-fat sour cream

2 ounces (about ¼ cup) plain whole-milk vanilla yogurt, preferably goat's milk yogurt

¼ teaspoon almond extract

2 tablespoons sliced almonds, lightly toasted

Light a medium-hot fire in a barbecue grill or preheat the broiler. Cut the peaches in half and remove the pits; no need to peel.

In a small saucepan, bring the vinegar and brown sugar to a boil, stirring to dissolve the sugar. Remove from the heat.

In a small bowl, blend the sour cream, yogurt, and almond extract.

Brush the peaches with the balsamic glaze and grill, or broil about 4 inches from the heat, turning and brushing 2 or 3 more times, until they are just slightly softened and have light brown grill marks. Remove to shallow bowls, allowing 2 halves per serving.

Drizzle about 2 teaspoons of the remaining balsamic glaze over each peach and top with 2 tablespoons of the almond cream. Garnish each serving with a sprinkling of toasted almonds.

Flourless Chocolate Roll with Banana Cream

There's no way to make a small one of these, so consider this a dinner party showstopper. Leftovers can be wrapped well and eaten the next day; they will still be delicious, even if the consistency is not perfect.

---

4 ounces bittersweet chocolate, chopped

5 eggs, separated

⅓ cup granulated sugar

1½ teaspoons vanilla extract

¾ cup heavy cream

¼ cup confectioners' sugar

1 tablespoon unsweetened cocoa powder

1 banana, very thinly sliced

Preheat the oven to 350°F. Line a 14 by 11-inch jelly roll pan with waxed paper or parchment. Butter the paper.

In a double boiler or a small heavy saucepan, melt the chocolate with 2 tablespoons of water over low heat, stirring until smooth. Remove from the heat.

Beat the egg yolks lightly. Gradually beat in the granulated sugar and continue to beat until the mixture forms a slowly dissolving ribbon when the whisk or beater is lifted, 2 to 3 minutes. Beat in the melted chocolate and 1 teaspoon of the vanilla.

In a large clean bowl with clean, dry beaters, whip the egg whites until stiff and glossy but not dry. Stir about one-fourth of the egg whites into the chocolate mixture. Scrape the remaining beaten egg whites into the bowl and fold into the chocolate mixture.

Turn the batter onto the lined pan and bake until the tip of a small knife inserted into the center comes out clean, about 15 minutes. Transfer to a rack, cover with a slightly damp kitchen towel, and let cool for about 20 minutes.

Beat the cream with 2 tablespoons of the confectioners' sugar until fairly stiff. Beat in the remaining ½ teaspoon of vanilla.

Arrange 2 large sheets of parchment or waxed paper on the counter, overlapping slightly. Gently lift off the towel and dust the top of the cake with the remaining 2 tablespoons of confectioners' sugar and the cocoa powder. Invert it onto the parchment, dusted side down. Spread the sweetened whipped cream over the cake, dot with the banana slices, and roll up snugly from one long side, using the parchment to help lift the cake. Cover and refrigerate for up to 4 hours before serving.

Strawberry-Banana Cream Pie

8 SERVINGS | 11 POINTS EACH

Yummy and creamy, this luscious dessert is low in calories, but because of the number of carbs, we consider it a splurge—one of those treats to be enjoyed once or twice a week.

1½ cups quartered fresh strawberries, plus 2 or 3 berries, halved or sliced, for garnish

1¼ cups coarsely mashed ripe banana (about 3 bananas)

¼ cup raw cane sugar

1 teaspoon vanilla extract

½ teaspoon almond extract

10 ounces (about 1¼ cups) plain whole-milk yogurt, preferably goat's milk yogurt

2 ounces reduced-fat cream cheese (Neufchâtel)

1 (0.25g) packet unflavored gelatin, dissolved in 2 table-spoons boiling water and cooled slightly

1 prepared 9-inch graham cracker crust

In a food processor or blender, combine the quartered strawberries, banana, sugar, vanilla, and almond extract. Pulse until the fruit is coarsely chopped. Add the yogurt, cream cheese, and dissolved gelatin and process until just blended.

Scrape the strawberry-banana cream filling into the prepared pie shell. Cover tightly with plastic wrap and refrigerate until firm, at least 3 hours, or overnight.

Just before serving, garnish with the reserved sliced berries.

CHAPTER 10

MOVE IT OR LOSE IT: HOW EXERCISE CAN IMPROVE BLOOD SUGAR

THOSE OF YOU WHO have read *The Acid Reflux Solution*, our book about healing heartburn naturally, know that I have always been challenged by my weight. I grew up an overweight little boy who had to wear those embarrassing husky pants that were reserved for chubby kids. In high school I was academically outstanding, but heck, the only team I belonged to was the debate team. I was not a jock. I did not participate in any sport. Lack of exercise was definitely one of the factors that contributed to my being overweight.

That all changed toward the end of my senior year in high school, when I became very interested in tennis. (I lived in South Florida, where the sun shines year round.) My friends and I all wanted to be tennis champions. By the summer before college, I was playing six to eight sets of tennis a day. Now, when I think back to that time, I can hardly imagine how I did it. Playing all those sets in the hot, muggy Florida sun is something that I could not possibly do today. But when you are nineteen years old, the body can withstand almost anything. Slowly but surely, my excess weight melted off. By the time I entered college, I had lost almost forty pounds.

While in college, I started swimming laps at the University of Miami's Olympic-size pool. In medical school, I joined the aerobics craze that was rampant in the early 1980s; plus, I began to lift weights. And along with thirty of my medical school classmates, I practiced karate for four years. I remember how we used to hurry from anatomy class—still smelling of formaldehyde—to the makeshift dojo on the medical school campus. That physical activity not only helped me keep my weight down, but it also helped me think more clearly and handle the day-to-day stress of college and medical school.

The point of this story is that I chose sports and exercises that I enjoyed and that I could do easily. It wouldn't have made much sense for me to take up snow skiing in South Florida. If you pick a sport or physical activity that is cumbersome, way beyond your budget, or too far away from home, you will have defeated your purpose before you even begin. For a physical activity program to be successful, make it easy, make it pleasurable, and make it practicable.

As soon as I became more physically active, my diet became healthier. When I started exercising regularly, my hunger pangs were fewer and farther between. There is a very involved physiological reason for this, but suffice it to say that my insulin and cortisol levels normalized and my blood sugar levels were more even throughout the day. Exercise alone is not enough to normalize your blood sugar, but without doing any form of exercise, you stand less of a chance of controlling your diabetes.

Exercise is just as vital as diet for controlling prediabetes and type 2 diabetes. One is not more important than the other; both are absolutely essential for better health. Food gives you the raw materials your body needs to function properly, and physical activity provides the energy and the infrastructure that allows those materials to do their work. Exercise also has a very particular role in lowering blood sugar. Take a look at these interesting facts:

- People with type 1 diabetes who measure out their insulin know that before a long, strenuous exercise session, they need to reduce their dose.

- A survey of 32,000 adult men followed for more than eighteen years recorded the fact that although 7 percent developed diabetes by the end of the study, those who spent an average of just over twenty minutes a day doing a mix of aerobic and weight-bearing exercise were 59 percent less likely to end up with the disease. This shows that exercise is associated with a decreased progression to diabetes.

- While the Institute of Medicine recommends Americans get at least thirty minutes of aerobic exercise every day, recent studies have shown that even if that time is broken up into ten- or fifteen-minutes intervals, it is helpful for cardiovascular health. If it is difficult to find the time, or you are too tired, you can divide your daily exercise into manageable portions.

As you probably know already, there are two different types of exercise: aerobic, which gives your heart and lungs a workout, and resistance, or weight training, which builds muscles and contributes to healthy bones. Both of these are beneficial for everyone, but they offer special gains to anyone with diabetes in a number of ways.

Because it is so vital that the muscles receive the energy they need during strenuous activity, any vigorous exercise, especially movement of the arms and legs, opens up a sort of back-door channel that allows glucose to flow from the blood into the skeletal muscles without any action of insulin. So even if you don't take insulin, repetitive movement—as in walking, running, cycling, swimming, or even dancing—helps lower blood sugar naturally. And vigorous exercise makes the use of your blood glucose as fuel much more efficient.

The cells that line our blood vessels produce a chemical called nitric oxide, which maintains the vessels' suppleness and allows them to expand as needed, keeping blood pressure under control. High blood pressure is frequently associated with type 2 diabetes, and it increases the damage to the microvessels as well as the risk of stroke. As we age, we produce less nitric oxide. Stimulation of the blood vessels by the rush of blood during aerobic exercise increases the production of nitric oxide and lowers blood pressure. Some studies show that regular exercise also reduces cholesterol levels.

Whatever sort of physical activity you choose, it's important to know that not all exercise is alike. Basically, you'll benefit most from a combination of strength training, which builds muscles, and aerobic training, which gets your heart pumping to strengthen your lungs and your cardiovascular system.

AEROBIC EXERCISE

Aerobic exercise is by definition physical activity performed in the presence of oxygen in the tissues. For our purposes, think of it as the type of exercise that makes your heart rate go up and makes you sweat. It causes the body to burn carbohydrates for fuel, which it gets first from energy stored in the muscles and later from the breakdown of fat. But you don't have to run an Olympic-quality sprint to be doing aerobic exercise. Light and moderate steady activity over time is aerobic, and it is most effective when performed at 60 to 85 percent of your maximum heart rate. Your heart rate is the same as your pulse: the number of times your heart beats in a minute.

Maximum heart rate is the fastest your heart can beat without risking damage. Most doctors recommend that a healthy individual not exceed 85 percent of his maximum heart rate. If you have any physical issues, you should ask your doctor to suggest a safe maximum heart rate for you. In fact, if you have been sedentary for many years or if you've had any cardiovascular or pulmonary issues, it's best to check with your doctor before beginning a new exercise program. You might get the go-ahead with a phone call, or a stress test may be recommended. It's always better to be safe than sorry. The American Diabetes Association recommends that anyone who has had diabetes for ten years or longer get a stress test before starting an exercise program.

Although there are more sophisticated formulas, an easy way to calculate maximum heart rate is to take 220 and subtract your age. Most treadmills have a way to measure heart rate, or you can buy an inexpensive apparatus that attaches to your chest or your wrist that will measure it for you. After you've been following your program for a while, you'll become familiar with how an increased rate feels and how it affects your body.

For many of us, however, maximum heart rate is a little like the top of Mt. Everest. We can look up at it, but we're probably not ever going to get there—or not for a very long while, anyway. It doesn't matter. Whatever you do that improves on where you are now (which might well be in a lounge chair) is going to increase your cardiovascular health, especially if you do it regularly. Keep in mind, even just walking ten to fifteen minutes straight, twice a day, is beneficial compared to being completely sedentary.

Walking is excellent for cardiovascular health. For people who are new to physical activity, it can be the best way to start. And you can do it indoors on a treadmill or outdoors on pavement or a country path, or even

Walking is an easy form of exercise, but it does carry the risk of falling. And for people with type 2 diabetes, this risk can be increased because of loss of vision, loss of sensation on the bottom of the feet, and cognitive decline, which could lead to missteps. This is something of a catch-22, because an analysis of more than fifty studies of older adults showed that a combination of exercise and vitamin D supplementation led to a 17 percent reduction in falls. Needless to say, developing the muscles in your legs and trunk as well as strengthening your bones will help prevent falls. But be sensible and do only what you and your physician assess as safe.

Most falls prevention programs recommend sturdy shoes with arch and ankle support. Nutrition is an especially important component in preventing falls, because proper nutrition keeps muscles and nerves healthy. Get enough calcium and protein as well as vitamins A, D, C, and K for muscle and bone health and B_6 and B_{12} for cognition. But always keep in mind that while supplements may be helpful if your diet is deficient, especially in vitamin D, it's always best to get your nutrients from your food. If you do take supplements, remember, more is not better; in fact, it can be damaging. Do not exceed recommended doses. And that means adding what you are getting from your multivitamin, if you're taking one, to the vitamins and minerals you are getting from your food.

inside the mall. Some studies recommend increasing the distance you walk in lots of little ways: park your car as far out in the lot as you can at work or at the mall, rather than jockeying for the closest spot. Take the stairs at work when you can. Set an alarm and get up from your desk and walk around for about five minutes every hour.

Wearing a simple pedometer can be great incentive for walking. Ideally, the goal is ten thousand steps per day, which is five miles, but I tell my patients to aim for five thousand at the beginning. You'll probably be doing at least one thousand to two thousand steps when you begin. Don't forget, every step counts—up and down the stairs, to the bathroom, to the refrigerator, walking the dog . . . Most pedometers clip onto a belt or can be slipped into a pocket. Some even connect to your computer.

At first, just wear the pedometer and go about your business as you would normally for three days. Then add up the totals and divide by three to get your average at baseline. Now, every two or three days, consciously increase your base activity level by fifty steps. You'll be surprised at how fast this adds up—to lots more steps and a healthier you.

What If I Hate the Gym?

Some of us groove on the scent of sweat and the sound of grunts and groans. Some of us are grossed out. Not all of us like to take our clothes off in front of strangers or, especially if we are obese, to parade up and down in clinging, sweaty clothes. Physical activity does not have to mean the gym. First of all, more exercise and yoga classes are being tailored for overweight individuals. Second, there are many more ways to be active than treadmills and machines.

Walking outside, walking your dog, walking the mall, doing yoga or tai chi, dancing, swimming, playing tennis or golf, gardening, doing active housework—every kind of active movement counts. What's important to avoid is sitting, especially for long stretches at a time.

What If I Can't Walk?

If you weigh more than 200 pounds, there is a good chance the pressure put on your joints has taken a toll on your knees, not to speak of the strain on your heart. I have many patients who report huffing and puffing just moving painfully from one side of the room to another. They can't stand long enough to cook their food, let alone try to indulge in physical activity.

Well, you have to start somewhere. So along with a serious diet, ideally supervised by a registered dietitian nutritionist, you have to begin moving. Seated arm and trunk exercises are one way. Many senior centers have chair yoga classes. Water aerobics is another highly recommended way, as it takes all the strain off your limbs. Some of these same programs may be helpful for people with severe peripheral neuropathy who are unsteady on their feet.

Whatever you do, keep at it and be patient with yourself. As you progress, keep moving the bar up. You'll be surprised at how far you can go over time if you remain patient and diligent. Eventually, you may move on to more strenuous exercise, and it's going to feel great!

ANAEROBIC EXERCISE

Anaerobic exercise is the same as resistance training. It takes place with forms of activity that stress muscles in short, intense bursts and is fueled by metabolic pathways that do not use oxygen. This type of exercise produces lactic acid, which is what makes muscles sore. You've heard the saying "No pain, no gain." Well, this is meant literally, though if you work out properly, you'll experience just a pleasant mild burn. And stretching both before and after can help minimize lactic acid buildup as well as decrease the risk of muscle strain.

Resistance training builds muscle tissue. Muscle is important for people with prediabetes and type 2 diabetes because it is metabolically active. Muscles constantly require fuel. And as mentioned earlier, skeletal muscle cells can suck the sugar out of your blood and help you burn fat, too. It's the metabolic action of muscles rather than the actual number of calories you burn that makes such a difference.

Contrary to popular lore, unless you're running marathons or biking thirty miles a day, you are not burning enough calories to lose substantial amounts of weight through exercise alone. The truth is that if you build muscle by doing anaerobic exercise, your basal metabolic rate will increase. That is to say, you will be burning more calories without even trying. Anaerobic exercise is an excellent way to avoid putting on more weight and to make your tissues more metabolically active. As a result, your body's furnace will be burning more calories. Have you ever noticed that once someone builds a lot of muscle he rarely becomes overweight again? He has found the secret: making the furnace bigger by putting on muscle mass.

Weight lifting, yoga, and sprinting are three forms of anaerobic exercise. It's unlikely you're going to be sprinting much, so I'm going to concentrate on the first two. When we speak of weight lifting, we're not talking about 50-pound barbells. For beginners and people without a lot of muscle strength, there are 2-pound and 5-pound weights that are all you need to begin. Some people prefer kettle bells, which are gripped a little differently. And of course there are the machines you see in the gym, which guide weight lifting within prescribed physical parameters. If you are going to start a weight-training regimen, I recommend that you get a trainer who can teach you how to safely lift the weights. If you have never lifted weights, I suggest you start with the machines before moving to free weights. It will be easier and safer for your body. You can move up to free weights once you build up some strength and understand how to lift with proper form.

Once you start lifting weights you will be exposed to a whole new world. Some people just want to get "big," meaning they want to develop big muscles. This is not your goal. Your goal is to lose body fat and gain a small amount of muscle tone. When you first begin a weight-lifting routine, alternate the regions of the body that you focus on; for example, do upper body on one day and lower body a couple of days later. Weight lifting (or strength training) builds muscle by putting enough demand and stress on the muscles to cause microscopic tears that the body responds to by both repairing and increasing the muscle. So be sure to leave a day in between those workouts for your body to rebuild the tissues it has torn down. Concentrate on the large muscle groups in the legs and trunk. But, as with most activities, start slow and low and work your way up.

No matter what kind of weight training you do, we strongly recommend that you start by working with a trainer, preferably someone who is not only experienced with exercise but is also certified at physical rehabilitation. Form is extremely important for weights—both for safety and for developing muscle mass with the greatest efficiency. A good trainer can teach you how to lift without hurting yourself and can both guide your form and tell you when you are ready to advance. Technically, the machines guide your form, because they have a limited range of motion, but not everyone has a body size and shape that is ideal for the machines. Even just a few sessions with a trainer and then refreshers every couple of months will help greatly.

Yoga is another great form of exercise. Although it doesn't involve lifting weights, it employs what is called *isometrics*, meaning the weight you're lifting is your own. Many yoga postures build strength and flexibility with the added bonus that the deep breathing helps draw oxygen into your tissues and encourages a meditative state at the same time. The gentle stretching increases circulation, which aerates the muscles. Relaxation is an added bonus.

MIXING IT UP

We've already explained the benefits of the two major types of exercise: aerobic and anaerobic, also known as resistance or weight training. The best overall exercise program mixes up the two for a full week of varied activity. Maybe you start by walking on five days and yoga on the other two days. Or you might have a routine where you lift weights at the gym every other day, walk on the days you're not at the gym, and take a water aerobics class on Sunday mornings. Or maybe you get all of your aerobic activity by briskly walking or jogging with your dog twice a day, and then add some weight training or other anaerobic activity a few times a week.

Keep in mind that these are schedules to work up to. Don't be discouraged if you start from a lower baseline. I certainly did when I entered high school. Maybe weight training for you means lifting a couple of 2-pound soup cans over your head. (Raising your arm to click the remote while you're planted in front of the television does not count as physical activity.) Any active movement is an improvement over being completely sedentary. And all physical activity, whether it's playing tag with your children, throwing a Frisbee on the beach with friends, or even cleaning out the garage counts toward improving your health.

CHAPTER 11

HOW STRESS AND SLEEP AFFECT TYPE 2 DIABETES

L IFE IS STRESSFUL; so what else is new? The economy, the kids, your weight, the mortgage, your weight, the bills, your job, your weight. And who gets a full night's sleep these days? Commutes are so long, downtime is so short, and both the TV and the computer are mesmerizing. *Get real! How could these facts of life possibly affect my diabetes?* you ask.

Well, it's always something. And in the case of type 2 diabetes, there are two things that are detrimental to improving your condition: too much stress and not getting enough sleep. One major way these both impact your diabetes is related to obesity. As you'll read, both unrelenting stress and chronic sleep deprivation lead to weight gain. But there are other effects, as well. Understanding how these impact your body may encourage you to improve at least one, if not both. Because as with diet and physical activity, these are two more ways you can seize control over factors that affect your health.

And they are not insignificant. Integrative medicine is becoming more and more prominent, because the way we have traditionally practiced has not led to a healthier population. We've come to realize that it's important to address the whole person, not just a bunch of lab tests. And why a person is stressed or doesn't sleep is part of that picture.

STRESS

When we're stressed, we release a hormone called *cortisol*. It's a key element in the flight-or-fight response, which is a phrase you may have heard. This natural response is our first line of protection against danger. Let's say *Tyrannosaurus rex* is approaching—thud, thud, thud. Are you going to run—fast—or stand your ground, pick up a wooden spear, and prepare to fight? I know which of those options I'd choose. But either way, you need extra physical resources to save yourself: extra energy, extra speed, and extra strength. You've probably heard some extraordinary stories about people lifting an enormous weight, like a car off a trapped child, in order to save a life. Evolution has given us this extra "zing" when we need it.

Our adrenaline surges, stimulating a chain reaction of hormones, which end up releasing cortisol. Cortisol, in turn, boosts our blood pressure and raises the amount of sugar in our blood. This slows our digestive metabolism, so if you had to, you could run for hours—well, longer than usual—and not get hungry, so you wouldn't need to slow down to eat. This is our body's way of ensuring we have enough sugar in our blood— the energy to do what needs to be done for survival. The flight-or-fight response preserves the energy you have during this critical period of survival while heightening your physical powers.

The problems arise when cortisol is pumped out not just in response to danger, but constantly, in response to the day-to-day stress of living. Chronically high blood pressure can ensue, which is problematic because it can lead to cardiovascular damage and even stroke. And we already know that people with type 2 diabetes are much more susceptible to these physical ills.

At the same time, having our blood sugar hormonally boosted this often is associated with insulin resistance and weight gain, leading to metabolic syndrome (see page 41). If you are also obese, you greatly increase your chances of developing both insulin resistance and type 2 diabetes. And stress often leads to lack of sleep, which encourages weight gain. It's something of a vicious circle.

So what can you do about managing ongoing day-to-day stress? Many things, but first of all you have to acknowledge that stress is a problem.

- Notice changes in the kinds of foods you choose to eat when you're tense. Some people find sugary foods; starchy, refined carbohydrates; and crunchy, fatty foods to be comforting.

- Notice how often or how inappropriately you get angry at family and friends when you are stressed out. Anger boosts your heart rate and blood pressure, stressing your cardiovascular system, and it pumps up your blood glucose as it readies your body for action.

- Notice whether stress and worry make you lose sleep. Specific life problems and generalized worry or depression often make it hard to fall asleep or stay asleep, which greatly affects your mood the next day. As we'll learn a little later in this chapter, lack of sleep also contributes to weight gain.

- Notice whether stress makes you act in a self-destructive fashion. Sometimes if we're overwhelmed, we just throw our hands up and say, *what's the difference?* Alcohol, drugs, fattening foods, five hours in front of the TV . . . Well, if you have type 2 diabetes, what you do and what you eat make a huge difference.

- What other ill effects do you notice from stress? Everyone is individual, and each person responds differently. Do you get hungry or lose your appetite? Do you get a headache or a stomachache? Do you tend to run away from your problems and avoid doing what you know you should to improve your health when you are stressed?

Once you identify the role stress plays in your life, it's important that you tease out which triggers are the most critical for you and find a way to manage them. Are your greatest sources of worry financial, emotional, or physical, problems with your children or spouse, loneliness, substance abuse, an addiction? Life is hard these days, and many of us experience more than one form of stress.

The next step is to become proactive. Simply making an effort to take control will automatically take the tension down a notch. And while you investigate other, more direct forms of dealing with your specific problems, you can start with diet and exercise. You know by now that eating the right nutrients improves your mood and helps you lose weight.

And I'll say it again: losing just 5 to 7 percent of your current body weight will improve your blood sugar levels and usually your blood pressure as well. You also know that physical activity boosts mood, lowers blood pressure, improves quality of sleep, and, if practiced regularly and vigorously enough, can improve cholesterol as well as blood sugar levels and improve cardiovascular health.

The following are some of the most common stressors and some ideas to explore for possible solutions. Go ahead and use our list as a starting point, or sit down and make your own list, then spend some quality time designing your own solutions. Putting yourself in charge will do you a world of good. And don't be afraid to ask others for help or ideas.

Weight and Health

I put these two together because they are inextricably linked. Being overweight or obese is a problem that can be daunting. And the more pounds you put on, it seems, the harder they are to lose and especially to keep off. It's essential you realize that eating the right foods really *can* make a difference with your mood and your health, especially if you have prediabetes or type 2 diabetes. But very few can go it alone. Studies have proven that ongoing counseling makes all the difference in the world. With a diagnosis of prediabetes or type 2 diabetes, you need an individualized plan for medication structured by your physician and an eating plan from a registered dietitian nutritionist and follow-up counseling.

The good news is that with the Affordable Care Act, many insurance plans now include overweight or obesity counseling with a registered dietitian nutritionist in their covered benefits. And diabetes is almost always covered. So if you have insurance that will pay for such counseling, take advantage of those wellness benefits. If you don't have such insurance coverage, check out diabetes self-management education courses, which are extremely reasonable at some pharmacies and public health departments. They are a must for anyone who is diagnosed with diabetes.

Finances

These are tough times. If you're up to your eyeballs in credit card debt, don't try to go it alone. Find a good financial advisor who can help you consolidate your debt. Many times your credit card company will work with you to help you pay off your debt over a longer period of time. So will the government. Then you have to put yourself on a really strict budget so you don't pile on even more debt.

If things are really critical and you're out of work, look to any social services you can. There are state, federal, and local services as well as churches and private food banks. Again, don't try to go it alone. Just reaching out will make you feel better.

Substance Abuse

Whether to alcohol, drugs, or obsessive gambling or shopping, all addictions are highly stressful. The motivation to change has to come from within you, but we all need support and professional help to overcome serious compulsions like this. Many established organizations with proven track records, like Alcoholics Anonymous, Alanon, and Gamblers Anonymous, are easy to access. If you prefer more privacy, you might look for an appropriate psychologist or counselor. Don't be shy about turning to your primary care practitioner for help or referrals to groups in your area. State and city public health departments may have programs or referrals.

Emotional Issues

There may well be a psychological component to your eating, especially if you are severely obese. Know that there is nothing weak about seeing a psychotherapist or psychologist. Most insurance plans cover more mental health than ever, even if you are on Medicare. Your local clergy may also offer supportive counseling. Venting to friends can help relieve pressure, but a professional will do a lot more to offer you permanent guidance as well as medication if you need it. Don't hesitate to start the process of getting help with your primary care doctor.

Work Problems

Anxiety about our professional lives is a major problem in modern life. Getting and keeping a job, dealing with difficult bosses, rising in the hierarchy or not—these are really tough issues to deal with, and they require patience. In this marketplace, you cannot just quit a job you do not like. So step back, assess the situation, and try to work out a plan of either calm confrontation or avoidance—whichever will do more to reduce the tension and put you in a more comfortable position.

Being a Caregiver

Now that so many parents work, the burden of caring for children has become much more stressful; time is in such short supply. Try to find an approved day care program to help out. Or involve your children in some of the chores you need to do. Rather than being simply a time-consuming duty, shopping and making dinner with your children can become a bonding experience or even a source of pride and pleasure.

At the same time, rates of Alzheimer's disease and other dementias are soaring as the population ages and especially with ballooning rates of diabetes, which contributes to the risk of cognitive decline in older adults. Helping your eighty-year-old father take a shower or feed himself is not

SIMPLE STRESS RELIEVERS

- Exercising
- Eating a proper diet
- Seeking counseling
- Being proactive about finding solutions to your problems
- Getting enough sleep
- Doing something nice for yourself
- Meditating
- Practicing yoga
- Having a massage
- Taking some private time for youself

something most of us were raised to do. Get help from social services, Alzheimer support groups, and hospice care, if necessary.

SLEEP

It turns out that your nocturnal downtime is not just a passive state. If you test your blood sugar with a finger stick in the morning, that reading will often be the highest of the day. (That's something to keep in mind when you're planning your meals.) Why is this the case? Because while you are obliviously at rest, your body thinks you are starving. After all, during the day, you feed it every three or four hours, and now it's not getting any nourishment for up to eight or ten hours. So while you sleep, your liver responds by manufacturing its own glucose in a process called *gluconeogenesis.*

At the same time, your body uses this rest period to refresh itself and put certain hormones in their proper balance. For some years, the question of whether lack of sleep caused weight gain was debated back and forth. It looked as if the evidence was about fifty-fifty. However, studies in recent years have convinced most researchers that habitually not getting enough sleep often enhances obesity and both increases the risk of type 2 diabetes and makes the condition worse.

It's estimated that as many as a third of all adults in the United States are sleep deprived. That means they are getting less than six hours of sleep a night. While sleep needs are partially genetically determined, most adults need at least seven or eight hours a night, and some require nine hours. One seven-and-a-half-year study of more than eighty thousand healthy adults, many of them older, found a strong correlation between getting less than five hours of sleep and excessive weight gain over time, regardless of their exact age, level of education, BMI, amount of physical activity, or whether or not they smoked. Other studies with younger populations have shown similar results.

Sleep deprivation—which usually means getting five hours of sleep or less—results in slower metabolic activity the next day. Levels of the stress hormone cortisol, as well as ghrelin, the hormone that tells us we're hungry, are elevated after insufficient rest. And morning blood glucose levels are also higher. Although all these hormonal regulations are still not completely understood, we do know that getting enough sleep tunes up our metabolic clock so that we function at peak efficiency the next day, and not getting enough sleep makes our glucose metabolism sluggish so that we expend fewer calories no matter what we do, which leads to weight gain and insulin resistance. And we know that both these factors are key in the development of prediabetes and type 2 diabetes.

Other studies have shown that being awake for those extra few hours when we should be sleeping often leads to obesity because if we're up, we get hungry. And if we're hungry, we make ourselves a little snack or a small meal—one we wouldn't have if we were sleeping. Even if you assume it's just a banana and a glass of milk, or half a peanut butter and jelly sandwich and a cup of tea, or perhaps a single glass of alcohol to help you relax, you're taking in enough calories to add a pound every two or three weeks.

How to Get Enough Sleep

You can get enough sleep if you take it seriously enough. Now that you know how important it is, make it a priority. Whatever you're doing, whatever stimulates you or stresses you out, try to put it away about an hour before you want to go to bed. Most sleep experts recommend no computer or TV in the bedroom and shades or curtains heavy enough to keep out light. Reduce sound as much as possible; if you live in a noisy community, consider buying a white noise machine to block it out. Make your bed a comfortable, cozy place to curl up in. Splurge on new pillows or a mattress if you need them. And turn down the thermostat. It will save on your heating bills, and most sleep experts recommend a slightly cooler temperature at night, with enough blankets or a comforter to suit your level of warmth.

Keep in mind that although many people think alcohol will put them to sleep, that's a misconception. While one glass of wine or a single cocktail earlier in the evening may be relaxing, too much alcohol will actually keep you awake. If you drink enough to sedate yourself, you may go under quickly, but you'll miss out on valuable REM sleep and will likely wake up with sweats or a headache in the middle of the night.

If you have trouble falling asleep or you wake up in the middle of the night, please do not ask your doctor for a sleeping pill. Because they supposedly clear the body quickly, these popular drugs are dispensed regularly. But the truth is, as they break down, the by-products these drugs produce make some people feel as if their brains are mashed potatoes for

hours. People report strange, often unconscious, and sometimes dangerous behaviors while they are supposedly sleeping. This includes driving a
car, walking outside, or preparing and eating a meal without realizing it.
And in the long term, some of these drugs are associated with higher inci-
dences of death from all causes.

To improve your chances of falling asleep, do not drink any caffeine
after 2:00 P.M. If you switch to tea later in the day, make sure it has no caffeine. Likewise with caffeinated sodas (which you shouldn't be drinking anyway) and energy drinks. Some people report they sleep better if they avoid
chocolate at night, because it is a trigger for acid reflux, which can wake up
susceptible individuals, and there is an alkaloid in chocolate that is a mild
stimulant.

Instead, go through the list of stress relievers we discussed earlier.
Also, ask your doctor whether you should be screened for obstructive sleep
apnea, or OSA. More than a third of obese adults suffer from sleep apnea, a
condition in which you literally stop breathing for seconds at a time, then
struggle to begin again. The result is that the body does not get all the oxygen it needs to do its housekeeping. Loud snoring is often an indication of
OSA. If you suffer from sleep apnea, you may wake up feeling unrefreshed
and may nod off during the day.

NATURAL SLEEPING POTION

A controlled trial in an assisted living facility for older adults, who often have
trouble falling asleep and staying asleep, found this mix to be helpful and safe.
All these ingredients can be purchased over the counter. That said, although
it is completely natural, because melatonin is a hormone and can interact with
hormone replacements and some psychoactive drugs, please check with your
health care provider before trying it. Also, any artificial sleep aid should be
considered helpful for anywhere from three days to three weeks. After that,
you should be in the habit of better sleep and should discontinue use.

About one hour before you want to fall asleep, take the following pills
with ½ cup of unsweetened applesauce or half an apple:

- 3 to 5 mg melatonin (depending upon your weight)
- 250 mg magnesium
- 15 mg zinc

Aim for going to bed earlier, because chances are you won't have the extra time in the morning except on the weekends. Give yourself a goal and work toward it, even if you get just an extra half hour.

If you have animals, make them sleep in their own beds. Even if the scene is peaceful when you doze off, dogs can stretch, run in their sleep, or try to push you off the bed in the middle of the night. And cats are nocturnal. When you want to get your sleep, they may decide it's a nice time to curl up on your head or chase an imaginary foe around the room.

Some people find that listening to meditation tapes before going to bed can help them fall asleep. Others find that reading will put them to sleep. If you have a snack in the evening, make it a small one, don't have too much protein, and don't drink too much fluid, which might cause you to wake up to pee in the middle of the night.

• • •

So here you have two other very real ways you can work to lower your blood sugar and your weight: find ways to reduce your stress, and get enough sleep. If you thought you were powerless over your diabetes, this chapter proves that you have some simple and empowering lifestyle choices to improve your health and manage your diabetes.

CHAPTER 12

BARIATRIC SURGERY: WHEN ALL ELSE FAILS

DURING MY MEDICAL CAREER there are two things that I have found the most difficult to treat and cure: obesity and drug addiction. Sometimes I wonder whether they are not one and the same. Indeed, many studies have recently demonstrated the addictive qualities of carbohydrates, especially sugar. I've seen thousands of patients over the past twenty-five years who promised me they would lose weight. Yet year in and year out, they don't lose an ounce. On the contrary, they usually end up gaining more weight over time.

The American Diabetes Association has made the following recommendation: "Bariatric surgery may be considered for adults with a BMI greater than 35 and type 2 diabetes, especially if the diabetes or associated comorbidities [other diseases] are difficult to control with lifestyle and pharmacological therapy."

My initial reaction to this recommendation, along with many of my colleagues, was that this is a bit drastic. However, considering the remote likelihood that many people will lose weight on their own, perhaps we do need to realize that in a certain segment of the population, taking a drastic measure to lose weight may be the only way to prolong life. Today, bariatric surgery is being recommended as an option to treat diabetes in the most obese patients who have failed both lifestyle changes and medications. However, there are risks associated with bariatric treatments, too.

I have a friend who became very despondent about his weight. During the course of his life he had tried many ways to lose weight, but he always gained it back, a pattern with which many of us are familiar. After much deliberation, he decided to undergo the gastric lap-band procedure. In this procedure, a band, which can be tightened or loosened, is placed around the outside of the stomach. It essentially cinches off part of the stomach, making the usable part of it smaller. You feel fuller quicker, eat less, and lose weight.

Although it sounds like a relatively simple way to battle your bulge, the truth about lap banding is that you do lose weight—perhaps 10 percent of your weight—but then you plateau. Most people learn to eat around the lap band. They eat more often, or they eat high-calorie soft foods (ice cream, anyone?). Unfortunately, lap banding usually does not create permanent weight loss. Most important, it does not change the mind-food relationship, which is the most important factor in permanent weight loss. In order to lose weight and keep it off, we must alter the way we think about food.

After the lap-band surgery, my friend was dissatisfied with the amount of weight he lost and wanted to lose more. So he decided to proceed with gastric bypass surgery. In gastric bypass, the stomach is stapled into a small pouch, and a part of the small intestine, where much of our nutrition is absorbed, is bypassed. This is a very serious surgery with many potential complications. It can cause chronic diarrhea and something called dumping syndrome caused by the intestine's being too short. It can also cause vitamin and mineral deficiencies because certain nutrients aren't being absorbed in large enough quantities.

On the other hand, gastric bypass can have tremendous advantages by drastically reducing weight in people who are at high risk for heart disease, stroke, and diabetes. My friend's case was much more complicated. Unfortunately, there were major complications during surgery and he ended up in cardiac arrest and had to have multiple surgeries to correct the complications of the initial surgery. He spent approximately four months in the hospital and was close to death on several occasions. Today he is doing well. He has to watch what and how he eats, but he is a new, happier man.

I don't share this case to scare you, but rather so you can see both the pluses and potential minuses of bariatric surgery. If you are a type 2 diabetic with a BMI of greater than 35 (see page 32) and you have *earnestly* tried to lose weight by modifying your diet and lifestyle without success, and you are also on medication, perhaps you should consider bariatric surgery. It's possible, too, that gastric lap-band surgery would help as a less drastic first measure. There are also inflatable balloons that can be placed temporarily in the stomach to make you feel full. Of course, all of these decisions should be discussed in detail with your health care provider before you decide on a course of action. But in the meantime, the following overview of pros and cons will give you a foundation to build on.

ADVANTAGES OF BARIATRIC SURGERY

There are many studies and analyses of people who have undergone bariatric surgery that show that it does work at normalizing blood sugar in diabetics. In one large comparison of more than three thousand diabetics who had undergone bariatric surgery, 78 percent reported remission of their diabetes. Remission was defined as normalization of blood glucose in the absence of medication. Plus, this effect was seen for more than two years.

Another study has shown that near or complete normalization of blood sugar was found in 45 percent to 95 percent of type 2 diabetics who underwent bariatric surgery. There is also evidence that bariatric surgery may affect diabetes not only by preventing the absorption of food, but also by stimulating a hormone called *incretin*. Incretin is a gastrointestinal hormone that increases the production of insulin in the pancreas. So bariatric surgery may work not only by decreasing the amount of food absorbed but also by causing your body to make more insulin to metabolize that food.

If we consider the cost of taking care of a diabetic, studies show that in the long run, bariatric surgery reduces the lifelong cost of therapy. Plus, with the knowledge that microscopic damage to organs is happening even in patients with prediabetes, bariatric surgery is a real option.

DISADVANTAGES OF BARIATRIC SURGERY

Although you've already heard about the complications that my friend had, death from bariatric surgery happens in less than 0.3 percent of cases. But there are other disadvantages as well as possible complications, including:

- Cost. Bariatric surgery is not often covered by insurance companies.
- Vitamin and mineral deficiencies, due to bypassing certain parts of the small intestine essential for their absorption.
- Osteoporosis, primarily due to calcium malabsorption.
- Hypoglycemia.
- Diarrhea.
- Nausea.
- Dumping syndrome. This is chronic diarrhea because the food you eat passes so quickly through your intestine (because it has been shortened) that there is not enough time to absorb the food. Therefore, much of it comes right out. Disgusting, right?
- Tiny meals. To maintain the weight loss and your health, for the rest of your life your meals have to be tiny.

Even though some studies show that morbidly obese diabetics who get bariatric surgery live longer than similar people who did not get the surgery, not all studies concur. There is no disagreement, however, that bariatric surgery is *not* the only solution. Lifelong lifestyle support and monitoring are still part of the treatment plan.

MY TWO CENTS

Most type 2 diabetes can be treated with diet and lifestyle changes. It is not easy, but it is not difficult, either. Before you embark on any lifestyle change, I recommend that you get honest about how much you're eating and moving. Ask yourself whether you really want to cure yourself of diabetes permanently (not whether you want to lose weight for a month, but permanently). Do you realize how your body is being destroyed by diabetes? Once you come to terms with these issues, then you're ready to commit to the Blood Sugar Budget program.

Before you officially get started, however, please make an appointment with your physician and begin our program with her guidance. I suggest that you give the program at least three months to see how it changes your A1C levels. If you also lose weight in the process, so much the better. (Oh, and you *will* lose weight.) I also suggest that you follow your physician's recommendations as to whether you require medications. If you need medications, embrace them. Remember, medications are not the problem—your diabetes is.

If, and only if, you are morbidly obese with a BMI of greater than 35 kg/m^2 (see page 32) *and* you have tried for two years to lose weight *and* you've become more active *and* even with medication your blood sugar level is not normalized, *then* you should consider bariatric surgery.

If there is one thing that my thirty years of being a physician has taught me, it's that there is no quick fix, but there are a lot of permanent solutions. *You* are your own permanent solution to treating diabetes. Believe in yourself. I do.

CHAPTER 13

THE DIABETES SOLUTION

S O AFTER READING all this material about diabetes, do you know what the solution is? The solution is *you:* You taking control of your health. You doing what you need to do to lower your blood sugar and reduce your risk of cardiovascular disease. You checking your blood sugar as needed to measure the effect of your meals and how you respond to certain foods. You partnering with your doctor and your nutritionist to do everything you can to fight the enemy: diabetes.

The Diabetes Solution is an integrative approach that uses everything we know about lowering blood sugar and improving health to prevent diabetes in the first place, return prediabetes numbers to normal levels, and manage type 2 diabetes. And by *manage,* we mean keeping complications to a minimum and jumping on any problems as they come up so they don't get any bigger.

FIRST THINGS FIRST

For starters, I hope you've learned the importance of screening—finding out your blood sugar numbers, especially your A1C, so that you know what kind of work is ahead of you. Once you pick up the challenge, the three biggest and most effective tasks are:

1. Lose weight! Losing just 5 to 7 percent of your current weight will make a huge difference in your A1C and your blood pressure, for starters.

2. Get moving. Find some sort of physical activity program you can stick with.

3. Work with your doctor to manage your medications. Don't be casual about it. If you have a prescription, you must take it religiously.

The Blood Sugar Budget will help you lose the weight you need to shed and lower your A1C. But it's not like taking a pill. It took you many years to get where you are. It's going to take you some months, at the least, to get where you need to go. Depending on your personality and other factors in your life, either dive right in or take the plan one step at a time, building up over a period of eight weeks, until you are on track. Then give yourself another two or three months to see the returns roll in.

Find some form of exercise or physical activity that works for you. Sure, a combination of aerobics and weight training offers the most benefit, but if you're so heavy that you can barely move across the room, just walking will be a huge step forward. Find an activity that is convenient, affordable, and pleasurable to you. It's the consistency that counts the most: at least thirty minutes a day, *every day.* Once you start getting in shape, you can build or add on to your activities.

In the meantime, let your doctor take care of you in any way necessary. Your medication may be needed simply to hold you over until you lose enough weight, or you may have a genetic tendency or an environmental issue that makes long-term meds a necessity. In either case, stay in touch with your physician. In addition to your regular check-ups, make another appointment if things change—for better or for worse. And if you have a diagnosis of diabetes, make a list of all the specialists you may need to see at least once a year, including:

- Ophthalmologist
- Podiatrist
- Dentist
- Cardiologist
- Nephrologist
- Neurologist

The sooner potential problems are assessed and addressed, the better the outcome. Reach out for help wherever you can get it.

AN INTEGRATIVE APPROACH

Integrative medicine looks at the entire person, not just one disease state. All right, you're working on your diet, exercise, and medications. But what else in your life is contributing to your diabetes? What stresses and problems are causing you to put on weight in the first place? Why can't you get a good night's sleep?

Feeling happier or more content, more at ease with yourself and more relaxed, will help you sleep at night and will improve your health. But it's certainly easier said than done. If you are having problems, all I can do is urge you to face them. You are not alone. These are tough times, and we're all going through it together. Reach out for the help you need, whether it be private therapy, group sessions, a religious or spiritual retreat, better

DIABETES SELF-MANAGEMENT EDUCATION

Remember, a structured diabetes self-management education program, which is usually reasonably priced and usually requires only three or four sessions, can remind you of everything we've gone over in this book. They're available at certified drugstores and public health departments. Many medical facilities and some doctors' offices have qualified diabetes educators who can present this standardized program, which was developed by the Diabetes Association of America. It's been proven that people who take these programs have lower average A1C than people who don't. You should take a class upon diagnosis, and every year or two after that to remind you of what you already know.

communication with your mate, moving closer to your family, furthering your education, or embarking on an adventure or new path in life.

The important thing is to be proactive. You'll feel better just knowing you are doing something to help yourself. And how incredible—of all the debilitating chronic diseases that we encounter, especially a little later in life, type 2 diabetes actually does respond to these very concrete lifestyle changes. Take it one step at a time, and always remember that doing something, no matter how small, is better than doing nothing.

Make yourself get up off that couch and turn off the television. Make yourself prepare a salad for lunch instead of going out for a burger and fries. Stop smoking! Stop drinking sweet beverages, whether they contain real sugar or artificial sweeteners, both of which are associated with obesity, which leads to diabetes.

IT'S NOT JUST ABOUT YOU

Forget about the staggering cost to the nation's health system related to diabetes: almost $175 *billion* per year! Forget the inconvenience, pain, and financial burden of dialysis (even though the government pays 80 percent). Ignore the hospital care, lost weeks and months of work, and devastation to your lifestyle if you've had an amputation. Not to speak of the decade of life you may be giving up. *What about your children?*

Remember, children learn as much or more from example as they do from teaching. What kind of a role model are you for your kids? If you're obese from eating a terrible diet, do you honestly think they're going to fare any better? I don't care if your mother and grandmother had diabetes. Is it just in your DNA, or do you practice a similar lifestyle to those female relatives: sedentary, with fattening foods and lots of refined carbohydrates? Experience has convinced many experts that health is largely 20 percent inherited genetic traits and 80 percent environmental factors *over which we have control!*

So go for it—you know you can do it. Follow *The Diabetes Solution* and the Blood Sugar Budget and see if you don't feel like a new person in three to six months. Drop me a line. I'd love to hear from you.

GLOSSARY

ADIPOSE TISSUE
The fat that is on our body.

ADRENALINE
Another word for epinephrine; one of the major fight-or-flight hormones that are expressed when we need a boost of energy or are under stress. It increases heart rate and raises blood glucose levels.

ADULT ONSET DIABETES
The name formerly used for type 2 diabetes, which is associated with obesity. It is not an autoimmune disease, and is usually non-insulin dependent. With increasing numbers of younger people developing the disease, the "adult onset" term is losing favor.

AEROBIC EXERCISE
A type of exercise that boosts heart rate and breathing (lung output), because it requires oxygen, such as jogging, bicycling, and swimming.

ALPHA-LIPOIC ACID (ALA)
A natural antioxidant, which also facilitates energy metabolism. Sometimes used as a supplement to improve insulin resistance and counter some symptoms of diabetes, such as numbness and tingling in the feet. Dark green vegetables, such as spinach and broccoli, are good dietary sources.

ALZHEIMER'S DISEASE
Neurological disease associated with fibrous protein tangles in the brain, which leads to dementia and eventually death. Diabetes increases the risk of all kinds of dementia, including Alzheimer's disease.

AMINO ACIDS
The building blocks of protein. Your body can manufacture many of them, but nine, which are called essential, must come from food.

ATHEROSCLEROSIS
A disease characterized by narrowing of the arteries due to a buildup of plaque. There is an increased risk of developing this so-called "hardening of the arteries" with diabetes.

AUTOIMMUNE DISEASE
Any disease where the body's immune system turns against itself and attacks its own cells as if they were foreign. Type 1 diabetes mellitus is an autoimmune disease where the immune system attacks the beta cells of the pancreas, thereby destroying the body's ability to make insulin, which is why it is sometimes called insulin-dependent diabetes.

BARIATRIC SURGERY
Surgery or surgical manipulation of the stomach and intestines, often performed to reduce weight. Several versions are lap banding, sleeve gastrectomy, and the most classic, roux-en-y, in which the stomach is stapled shut, leaving only a pouch the size of a fist, foreshortening and bypassing a length of the upper part of the small intestine. This type of surgery often cures diabetes immediately, but there are severe nutritional consequences and dietary restrictions for life.

BMI (BODY MASS INDEX)
A metric measurement of a person's weight in relation to his height squared, which offers an approximation of the proportion of the body that is made up of fat cells: 18.5 to 24.9 kg/m² is considered normal, 25 to 29.9 kg/m² represents overweight, and 30 kg/m² and up is considered obese. Both overweight/obese and underweight put people at higher risk for disease.

CALCIUM
A mineral essential for strong teeth and bones as well as muscle movement and nerve communication. It is also one of the major electrolytes and comprises the largest mineral reserve in the body. Dietary sources are dairy foods, fish, and dark leafy greens.

CALORIE
A unit of energy commonly used to measure the amount of energy ingested with food. Carbohydrates and proteins contain 4 calories per gram; fat contains 9 calories per gram, which is why fat cells offer the most efficient way to store energy for use in between meals.

CARBOHYDRATES
Produced by plants from the energy of the sun, carbohydrates are made up of hydrogen, oxygen, and carbon, which the body burns for fuel. Sugars and starches are two major carbohydrates.

CEREBRAL VASCULAR ACCIDENT (CVA)
Commonly known as a "stroke," a CVA is where an artery of the brain "bursts" and cannot deliver blood to its assigned area. As that area dies off due to lack of blood, it causes permanent damage to that area and the functions it controls. A CVA can cause paralysis, blindness, or inability to speak, depending on which part of the brain is affected. Diabetes increases the risk of CVA, but high blood pressure and cigarette smoking are the main causes of stroke.

CHOLESTEROL
A type of animal fat found in food. Too much cholesterol contributes to atherosclerosis and eventually to heart attacks and stroke. However, appropriate amounts of cholesterol in the diet are essential for producing sexual hormones and for the health of cell walls, which are vital for much of the communication that goes on within the body.

CHROMIUM PICOLINATE
A naturally occurring element that is associated in some cases with less insulin resistance. In areas of the world where chromium is missing from the soil, there are higher rates of diabetes.

COFACTOR
A molecule or chemical that increases the effectiveness or speed of a reaction.

CONGESTIVE HEART FAILURE
When the muscle tissues of the heart have been so extensively damaged that it cannot pump sufficient amounts of blood with each beat, leading to the eventual backing up of body fluids, manifesting in congested lungs and swelling of the extremities.

CORPUS CAVERNOSUM
One of the three chambers of the penis that must be filled with blood in order to achieve an erection.

CORTISOL
One of the so-called fight-or-flight hormones increased by stress. Cortisol increases blood glucose levels by increasing gluconeogenesis. Elevated cortisol levels over time have been associated with weight gain.

CURCUMIN
An extract of turmeric that has anti-inflammatory properties. A couple of small controlled trials showed that 750 mg of curcumin injested twice a day greatly reduced the number of people with prediabetes from advancing to diabetes.

DASH (DIETARY APPROACHES TO STOP HYPERTENSION) DIET
A healthful, very low sodium, low meat diet that has been proven to significantly lower blood pressure.

DEMENTIA
A descriptive mental condition that is associated with greater than normal forgetfulness and loss of mental acuity as well as inability to perform the tasks of daily living. Uncontrolled diabetes increases the risk of dementia.

DIABETES, TYPE 1
An autoimmune disease where destruction of the beta cells in the pancreas leads to loss of insulin production. This results in very high blood glucose levels and requires daily insulin supplementation to prevent death. Onset is usually in childhood and adolescence.

DIABETES, TYPE 2
A disease where decreased insulin production and/or decreased insulin sensitivity (the ability to use existing insulin effectively) leads to higher blood sugar levels. If not treated to lower blood glucose, many dangerous complications arise over time. May occur at any age, with a very high correlation with overweight and obesity. In most individuals, type 2 diabetes is highly responsive to diet, weight loss, and exercise.

DIALYSIS
An artificial mechanical cleansing of the blood made necessary because of kidney failure. Diabetes is the leading cause of end-stage kidney disease.

DUMPING SYNDROME
Rapid diarrhea that occurs after eating due to the gut's inability to completely absorb what has just been eaten. Often a result of the foreshortening of the intestine during bariatric surgery; can be managed and sometimes alleviated over time with proper diet. It is also associated with other symptoms that include sweating, nausea, and weakness followed by extremely urgent uncontrollable diarrhea.

EPINEPHRINE
Another word for adrenaline.

ERECTILE DYSFUNCTION
The inability to get or maintain an appropriate penile erection.

ESTRADIOL
Another name for estrogen, the primary female hormone that is produced from cholesterol and is responsible for feminizing characteristics.

FASTING BLOOD SUGAR
A test used to measure blood glucose levels after fasting (not eating or drinking any calories) for at least 8 hours. The test is often used to diagnose diabetes.

FAT

One of the three macronutrient food groups. Carbohydrate and protein are the other two. Fat is useful for storing energy and is essential for healthy functioning, but excess intake can lead to weight gain.

GESTATIONAL DIABETES (GDM)

A type of diabetes that can occur during pregnancy and disappear after delivery. If untreated, it can lead to babies who are too large, posing risk for the mother and future health of the child. Women who suffer from GDM are at greater risk of developing type 2 diabetes.

GLUCAGON

A hormone produced in the alpha cells of the pancreas and released into the bloodstream when blood sugar is too low. It boosts blood sugar by stimulating the liver to produce glucose and increasing the release of glucose from the liver into the blood while at the same time inhibiting the liver from storing glucose.

GLUCONEOGENESIS

The creation of glucose in the liver, either from stored glycogen or from dietary fats and proteins. It is necessary when the body has used up all of its stores of available energy or during starvation.

GLUCOSE

A one-molecule sugar that is the body's preferred source of energy and the brain's favorite food. Most other sugars and starches are quickly broken down into glucose by the digestive system.

GREHLIN

A gut hormone that signals to us when we are hungry and turns off when we have had enough to eat. When people are obese, this hormone is ineffectual.

HEART ATTACK

Clinically called a myocardial infarction (MI), heart attack is a common term used to describe chest pain and the death of heart tissue caused by poor blood flow to the heart.

HEMOGLOBIN A1C

A measure of the percentage of glucose that is bound to the surface of red blood cells. It correlates with the average blood glucose over a prior three months. An A1C measurement of 6.5 percent or higher is one of the definitions of diabetes.

HYPERGLYCEMIA

Elevated blood sugar, which is considered anything above 100 mg/dl.

HYPERTENSION

High blood pressure. Classic normal is no higher than 120/80 mm Hg. A reading of 120 to 139 over 80 to 89 signals prehypertension. High blood pressure begins at 140/90 mm Hg.

HYPOGLYCEMIA

Low blood sugar. Symptoms often include cold sweats, clamminess, and dizziness. The condition is dangerous because you could pass out and hurt yourself.

INSULIN

A hormone manufactured in the beta cells of the pancreas that lowers blood sugar by facilitating the movement of glucose from the bloodstream into the cells, muscles, and organs of the body to be used for energy.

INSULIN PUMP

A machine that continuously measures a person's blood sugar level and automatically administers the correct amount of insulin into his or her blood.

IRON

A mineral found in nature that is essential for manufacturing the red blood cell's hemoglobin. Hemoglobin is essential in carrying oxygen to all the cells of the body. Though vital, iron is highly toxic, so excess intake is discouraged.

KETOACIDOSIS

Acidification of the blood caused by excess ketones. Ketones are a by-product of using fat as the body's energy source. Ketones lower the pH of the blood into the acidic range. Having an acid blood pH can be deadly. Diabetics who are not on an effective treatment often have ketoacidosis because the body uses fat rather than glucose as the primary energy source.

KIDNEY FAILURE

The last stage of chronic kidney disease, which can be caused by diabetes. When the kidneys lose their ability to filter out toxins, maintain blood pressure, and establish proper acid/base balance in the body, the only resort is dialysis to preserve life.

LEPTIN

A hormone that tells us we have eaten enough—i.e., a signal of satiety—by being sensitive to the amount of fat, or energy, stored in the body. In the obese state, people are resistant to leptin in the same way they are resistant to insulin.

LIPIDS

Another word for fats. Usually referring to the fats floating in the blood— cholesterol and tryiglycerides, for example.

MEDITERRANEAN DIET

A dietary plan based on the eating habits of the countries around the Mediterranean region that have lower rates of many chronic diseases, including obesity, diabetes, heart disease, high blood pressure, and cancer. The diet emphasizes vegetables, fruits, whole grains, nuts, fish, and chicken rather than red meat and low-fat dairy.

MELATONIN

A naturally occurring substance that is associated with being able to sleep well. Supplementing your diet with melatonin may help insomnia. Lack of sleep has been associated with obesity, which in turn has been associated with type 2 diabetes.

METABOLIC SYNDROME

A group of symptoms, including abdominal obesity, high blood pressure, elevated triglycerides, and low HDL cholesterol that often—though not always—includes high blood sugar. Metabolic syndrome often leads to type 2 diabetes.

NEUROPATHY

Damage to nerves, which results in tingling or loss of sensation. Neuropathy of the hands and feet are often one of the first symptoms of diabetes.

NITRATES

Naturally occurring nitrogen-containing compounds that are often used to maintain the pink color in preserved and cured meats. In the stomach, nitrates are converted into nitrites, which are carcinogenic. Vitamin C, as in a glass of orange juice, can mitigate the effect of ingested nitrates.

NITRIC OXIDE

A gas produced by the lining of arteries and veins under certain conditions, such as aerobic exercise, which facilitates the relaxation of the blood vessels. A decrease in nitric oxide has been associated with erectile dysfunction.

OBESITY

An excessive and dangerous amount of body fat. Defined as having a BMI of greater than 30 kg/m^2.

ORAL GLUCOSE TOLERANCE TEST (OGTT)

One of the tests used to diagnose diabetes. In a fasting state the patient is asked to consume a measured amount of oral glucose. The blood sugar level is then measured over the next two hours. Elevated levels of blood sugar may be sufficient to diagnose whether the person has diabetes.

OSTEOPENIA

A state of reduced bone density that often leads to osteoporosis.

OSTEOPOROSIS
A pathological state of reduced bone density that can result in painful fractures and serious incapacitation.

PANCREAS
The organ tucked behind the stomach and the top of the small intestine, which releases many digestive hormones that help us digest our food properly. The pancreas also creates insulin.

POLYCYSTIC OVARIAN SYNDROME (PCOS)
A congenital endocrine disorder that is typified by enlarged ovaries infiltrated by many cysts, which leads to hyperandrogenism and insulin resistance. It is the most common reason for female infertility and shares many characteristics with metabolic syndrome.

PREDIABETES
A condition characterized by elevated blood sugar that is above normal but not yet fully diabetic. An A1C of between 5.6 and 6.5 indicates prediabetes.

PROTEIN
A large nitrogen-containing molecule made of amino acids that is essential for life. Our DNA determines which proteins different cells express, and these ultimately direct all the structures and functions of the body. Hormones and enzymes are proteins; much of our muscle tissue and many organs are also composed largely of protein. Dietary protein can be obtained from meat, poultry, fish, dairy, grains, and vegetables.

PSYLLIUM
A natural fiber often given as a supplement to improve bowel regularity and bind cholesterol, removing it from the body.

RESISTANCE TRAINING
Weight-bearing exercise that helps build muscle and bone. Having more muscle mass increases our basal metabolic rate.

RETINOPATHY
Disease of the retina (the "visual screen" of the eye) caused by damage to the many tiny blood vessels in the back of the eye. One of the first signs may be blurry vision. A common complication from diabetes.

STARCH
A carbohydrate composed of straight lines or webs of anywhere from three to tens of thousands of sugar molecules strung together. Bread, potatoes, pasta, and rice are common starches.

STROKE
See Cerebral Vascular Accident.

SUGAR

A general term referring to a type of carbohydrate. While there are many forms of sugar, the type we commonly refer to, which is our major form of sweetener, is table sugar, technically sucrose or dextrose, which is composed of two basic one-molecule sugars: glucose and fructose. The body uses sugar for energy; if there is too much, it is converted into fat.

TRIGLYCERIDE

The most common dietary fat as well as the type of fat the body uses for storage. It is composed of a glycerol molecule onto which three different fats are attached. To lose weight, this molecule has to be taken apart so that the carbon molecules can be burned for energy.

VITAMIN D

One of the naturally occurring fat-soluble vitamins, along with vitamins A, E, and K. Almost every cell in the body has receptors for vitamin D, so even though not all of its functions are known, the assumption is that it is very important. We do know that vitamin D is absolutely essential for the absorption of calcium. Studies are under way to determine whether supplementation can help prevent people with prediabetes from progressing to diabetes.

REFERENCES

Books

American Diabetes Association Complete Guide to Diabetes, 5th edition, by the American Diabetes Association, Alexandria, VA, 2011.

Dr. Bernstein's Diabetes Solution: The Complete Guide to Achieving Normal Blood Sugars, 4th revised updated edition, by Richard K. Bernstein. Little, Brown and Company, New York, 2011.

Glycemic Load Diabetes Solution by Rob Thompson, MD, recipes by Dana Carpender. McGraw-Hill Education, New York, 2012.

Nutrition and Diagnosis-Related Care, 8th edition, by Sylvia Escott-Stump. Lippincott Williams & Wilkins, Baltimore, MD, 2012.

The First Year: Type 2 Diabetes: An Essential Guide for the Newly Diagnosed, by Gretchen Becker and Allison B. Goldfine. Da Capo Press, New York, 2006.

Periodicals and Journals

Acheson KJ. Diets for body weight control and health. *European Journal of Clinical Nutrition.* 2013; 67:462–66.

Alhazmi A, Stojanovski E, McEvoy M, Garg ML. Macronutient intakes and development of type 2 diabetes: a systematic review and meta-analysis of cohort studies. *Journal of the American College of Nutrition.* 2012; 31(4).

American Diabetes Association. Standards of medical care in diabetes—2014. *Diabetes Care.* 2014 Jan; 37(Supp 1).

Asemi Z, Samimi M, Tabassi Z, Esmaillzadeh A. The effect of DASH diet on pregnancy outcomes in gestational diabetes: a randomized controlled clinical trial. *European Journal of Clinical Nutrition* 2014 Jan 15. doi: 10.1038/ejcn.2013.296. [Epub ahead of print].

Aune D, Norat T, Romundstad P, Vatten LJ. Dairy products and the risk of type 2 diabetes: a systematic review and dose-response meta-analysis of cohort studies. *American Journal of Clinical Nutrition.* 2013 Oct; 98(4):1066–83. doi: 10.3945/ajcn.113.059030. Epub 2013 Aug 14.

Babu PVA, Liu D, Gilbert ER. Recent advances in understanding the anti-diabetic actions of dietary flavonoids. *Journal of Nutritional Biochemistry.* 2013 Nov; 24(11):1777–89. doi: 10.1016/j.jnutbio.2013.06.003. Epub 2013 Sep 9.

Benedict C, Hallschmid M, Lassen A, Mahnke C, Schultes, Schioth HB, Born J, Lange T. Acute sleep deprivation reduces energy expenditure in healthy men. *American Journal of Clinical Nutrition.* 2011 June; 93(6):1229–36.

Black PH. The inflammatory consequences of psychologic stress: relationship to insulin resistance, obesity, atherosclerosis and diabetes mellitus, type II. *Medical Hypotheses.* 2006; 67:879–91.

Brown RJ, Walter M, Rother KI. Effects of diet soda on gut hormones in youths with diabetes. *Diabetes Care.* 2012 May; 35(5):959–64. doi: 10.2337/dc11-2424. Epub 2012 Mar 12.

Carter A, et al. Risk of incident diabetes among patients treated with statins. *British Medical Journal.* 2013 May; 345(f2610). doi: 10.1136/bmj.f2610.

Chang JS, You YH, Park SY, Kim JW, Kim HS, Yoon KH, Cho JH. Pattern of stress-induced hyperglycemia according to type of diabetes: a predator stress model. *Diabetes & Metabolism Journal.* 2013 Dec; 37(6):475–83. doi: 10.4093/dmj.2013.37.6.475. Epub 2013 Dec 12.

Chen F, Xiong H, Wang J, Ding X, Shu G, Mei Z. Antidiabetic effect of total flavonoids from Sanguis draxonis in type 2 diabetic rats. *Journal of Ethnopharmacology.* 2013 Oct 7; 149(3):729–36. doi: 10.1016/j.jep.2013.07.035.

Christensen AS, Viggers L, Hasselström K, Gregersen S. Effect of fruit restriction on glycemic control in patients with type 2 diabetes—a randomized trial. *Nutrition Journal.* 2013 Mar 5; 12:29. doi: 10.1186/1475-2891-12-29.

Chrysant SG, Chrysant GS. An update on the cardiovascular pleiotropic effects of milk and milk products. *Journal of Clinical Hypertension* (Greenwich). 2013 Jul; 15(7):503–10. doi: 10.1111/jch.12110. Epub 2013 Apr 29.

Corella D, Carrasco P, Sorlí JV, Estruch R, Rico-Sanz J, et al. Mediterranean diet reduces the adverse effect of the TCF7L2-rs7903146 polymorphism on cardiovascular risk factors and stroke incidence: a randomized controlled trial in a high-cardiovascular-risk population. *Diabetes Care.* 2013 Nov; 36(11):3803–11. doi:10.2337/dc13-0955.

Dalen JE, Devries S. Diets to prevent coronary heart disease 1957–2013: what have we learned? *American Journal of Medicine.* 2014 May; 127(5):364–9. doi: 10.1016/j.amjmed.2013.12.014.

van Dam RM, Naidoo N, Landberg R. Dietary flavonoids and the development of type 2 diabetes and cardiovascular diseases: review of recent findings. *Current Opinions in Lipidology.* 2013 Feb; 24(1):25–33. doi: 10.1097/MOL.0b013e32835bcdff.

Ding J, et al. Association between non-subcutaneous adiposity and calcified coronary plaque: from the multi-center MESA study. *American Journal of Clinical Nutrition.* 2008; 88:645–50.

Dunkler D, Dehghan M, Teo KK, et al. ONTARGET Investigators. Diet and kidney disease in high-risk individuals with type 2 diabetes mellitus. *JAMA Internal Medicine.* 2013 Oct 14; 173(18):1682–92.

Elwood PC, Gallacher J, Givens I, et al. The survival advantage of milk and dairy consumption: an overview of evidence from cohort studies of vascular diseases, diabetes and cancer. *Journal of the American College of Nutrition.* 2008 Dec; 27(6):7235–345.

Fagherazzi G, Vilier A, Sartorelli DS, Lajous M, Balkau B, Clavel-Chapelon F. Consumption of artificially and sugar-sweetened beverages and incident type 2 diabetes in the Etude Epidémiologique aupre's des femmes de la Mutuelle Genérale de l'Education Nationale–European Prospective Investigation into Cancer and Nutrition cohort. *American Journal of Clinical Nutrition.* 2013; 97:517–23.

Foster-Powell K, Holt S, Brandmiller JC. International table of glycemic index and glycemic load values: 2002. *American Journal of Clinical Nutrition.* 2002; 76:5–56.

German JB, Gibson RA, Krauss RM, Nestel P, Lamarche B, van Staveren WA, Steijns JM, de Groot LC, Lock AL, Destaillats F. A reappraisal of the impact of dairy foods and milk fat on cardiovascular disease risk. *European Journal of Nutrition.* 2009 Jun; 48(4):191–203. Epub 2009 Mar 4.

Gregg EW, Li Y, Wang J, Burrows NR, Ali MK, Rolka D, Williams DE, Geiss L. Changes in diabetes-related complications in the United States, 1990–2010. *New England Medical Journal.* 2014 Apr 17; 370:1514–23. doi: 10.1056/NEJMoa1310799.

Guzzetti C, Pilia S, Ibba A, Loche S. Correlation between cortisol and components of the metabolic syndrome in obese children and adolescents. *Journal of Endocrinological Investigation.* 2014 Jan; 37(1):51–6. doi: 10.1007/s40618-013-0014-0. Epub 2014 Jan 8.

Hauner H, Wolfram G, Bechthold A, et al. Evidence-based guideline of the German Nutrition Society: carbohydrate intake and prevention of nutrition-related diseases. *Annals of Nutrition and Metabolism.* 2012; 60 (suppl 1):1–58.

Hooper L, Kay C, Abdelhamid A, Kroon PA, Cohn JS, Rimm EB, Cassidy A. Effects of chocolate, cocoa, and flavan-3-ols on cardiovascular health: a systematic review and meta-analysis of randomized trials. *American Journal of Clinical Nutrition.* 2012 Mar; 95(3):740–51. doi: 10.3945/ajcn.111.023457. Epub 2012 Feb 1.

Hyun B, Shin S, Lee A, Lee S, Song Y, Ha NJ, Cho KH, Kim K. Metformin down-regulates TNF-α secretion via suppression of scavenger receptors in macrophages. *Immune Network.* 2013 Aug; 13(4):123–32. doi: 10.4110/in.2013.13.4.123. Epub 2013 Aug 26.

Jaudszus A, Kramer R, Pfeuffer M, Roth A, Jahreis G, Kuhnt K. Trans-palmitoleic acid arises endogenously from dietary vaccenic acid. *American Journal of Clinical Nutrition.* 2014 Jan 15; 99(3):431–5. doi: 10.3945/ajcn.113.076117.

Jennings A, Welch AA, Spector T, Macgregor A, Cassidy A. Intakes of anthocyanins and flavones are associated with biomarkers of insulin resistance and inflammation in women. *Journal of Nutrition.* 2014 Feb; 144(2):202–8. doi: 10.3945/jn.113.184358.

Jiang X, Zhang D, Jiang W. Coffee and caffeine intake and incidence of type 2 diabetes mellitus: a meta-analysis of prospective studies. *European Journal of Nutrition.* 2014 Feb; 53(1):25–38. doi: 10.1007/s00394-013-0603-x. Epub 2013 Oct 23.

Khavandi K, Amer H, Brownrigg J. Strategies for preventing type 2 diabetes: an update for clinicians. *Therapeutic Advances in Chronic Disease.* 2013 Sept; 4(5):242–61.

de Koning L, Malik VS, Rimm EB, Willett WC, Hu FB. Sugar-sweetened and artificially sweetened beverage consumption and risk of type 2 diabetes in men. *American Journal of Clinical Nutrition.* 2011 Jun; 93(6):1321–7. doi: 10.3945/ajcn.110.007922. Epub 2011 Mar 23.

Kratz M, Baars T, Guyenet S. The relationship between high-fat dairy consumption and obesity, cardiovascular, and metabolic disease. *European Journal of Nutrition.* 2013 Feb; 52(1):1–24. doi: 10.1007/s00394-012-0418-1. Epub 2012 Jul 19.

Krebs JD, Bell D, Hall R, Parry-Strong A, Docherty PD, Clarke K, Chase JG. Improvements in glucose metabolism and insulin sensitivity with a low-carbohydrate diet in obese patients with type 2 diabetes. *The Journal of the American College of Nutrition.* 2013 Feb; 32(1):11–7. doi: 10.1080/07315724.2013.767630.

Kris-Etherton PM, Grieger JA, Hilpert KF, West SG. Milk products, dietary patterns and blood pressure management. *The Journal of the American College of Nutrition.* 2009 Feb; 28(suppl 1):103S–19S.

Labazi H, Wynne BM, Tostes R, Webb RC. Metformin treatment improves erectile function in an angiotensin II model of erectile dysfunction. *The Journal of Sexual Medicine.* 2013 Sep; 10(9):2154–64. doi: 10.1111/jsm.12245. Epub 2013 Jul 24.

Labonté MÈ, Couture P, Richard C, Desroches S, Lamarche B. Impact of dairy products on biomarkers of inflammation: a systematic review of randomized controlled nutritional intervention studies in overweight and obese adults. *American Journal of Clinical Nutrition.* 2013 Apr; 97(4):706–17. doi: 10.3945/ajcn.112.052217. Epub 2013 Feb 27.

Larsson SC, Virtamo J, Wolk A. Dietary fats and dietary cholesterol and risk of stroke in women. *Atherosclerosis.* 2012 Mar; 221(1):282–6. doi: 10.1016/j.atherosclerosis.2011.12.043. Epub 2012 Jan 8.

Ma X, Zhu S. Metabolic syndrome, diabetes mellitus, cardiovascular and neurodegenerative diseases. *European Journal of Clinical Nutrition.* 2013; 67:518–21.

McGregor RA, Poppitt SD. Milk protein for improved metabolic health: a review of the evidence. *Nutrition & Metabolism* (London). 2013 Jul 3; 10(1):46. doi: 10.1186/1743-7075-10-46.

Mozaffarian D, Cao H, Hotamisligil GS. Trans-palmitoleic acid, metabolic risk factors, and new-onset diabetes in US adults. *Annals of Internal Medicine.* 2010 Dec 21; 153(12):790–9. doi: 10.7326/0003-4819-153-12-201012210-00005.

Mozaffarian D, Cao H, King IB, Lemaitre RN, Song X, Siscovick DS, Hotamisligil GS. Circulating palmitoleic acid and risk of metabolic abnormalities and new-onset diabetes. *American Journal of Clinical Nutrition.* 2010 Dec; 92(6):1350–8. doi: 10.3945/ajcn.110.003970. Epub 2010 Oct 13.

Mozaffarian D, de Oliveira Otto MC, Lemaitre RN, Fretts AM, Hotamisligil G, Tsai MY, Siscovick DS, Nettleton JA. Trans-palmitoleic acid, other dairy fat biomarkers, and incident diabetes: the Multi-Ethnic Study of Atherosclerosis (MESA). *American Journal of Clinical Nutrition.* 2013 Apr; 97(4):854–61. doi: 10.3945/ajcn.112.045468. Epub 2013 Feb 13.

Nagata C, Nakamura K, Wada K, Tsuji M, Tamai Y, Kawachi T. Branched-chain amino acid intake and the risk of diabetes in a Japanese community: the Takayama Study. *American Journal of Epidemiology.* 2013 Oct 15; 178(8):1226–32. doi: 10.1093/aje/kwt112. Epub 2013 Sept 5.

Nathan DM, Davidon MB, DeFronzo RA, Henry RR, Pratley R, Zinman B. Impaired fasting glucose and impaired glucose tolerance: implications for care. *Diabetes Care.* 2007 Mar; 30(3):753–9. doi: 10.2337/dc07-9920.

Nestel PJ, Mellett N, Pally S, Wong G, Barlow CK, Croft K, Mori TA, Meikle PJ. Effects of low-fat or full-fat fermented and non-fermented dairy foods on selected cardiovascular biomarkers in overweight adults. *British Journal of Nutrition.* 2013 Dec; 110(12): 2242–9. doi: 10.1017/s0007114513001621. Epub 2013 Jan 12.

Nestel PJ, Straznicky N, Mellett NA, Wong G, De Souza DP, Tull DL, Barlow CK, Grima MT, Meikle PJ. Specific plasma lipid classes and phospholipid fatty acids indicative of dairy food consumption associate with insulin sensitivity. *American Journal of Clinical Nutrition.* 2014 Jan; 99(1):46–53. doi: 10.3945/ajcn.113.071712. Epub 2013 Oct 23.

de Oliveira Otto MC, Mozaffarian D, Kromhout D, Bertoni AG, Sibley CT, Jacobs DR Jr, Nettleton JA. Dietary intake of saturated fat by food source and incident cardiovascular disease: the Multi-Ethnic Study of Atherosclerosis. *American Journal of Clinical Nutrition.* 2012 Aug; 96(2):397–404. doi: 10.3945/ ajcn.112.037770. Epub 2012 Jul 3.

Onitilo AA, Stankowski RV, Berg RL, Engel JM, Glurich I, Williams GM, Doi SA. Type 2 diabetes mellitus, glycemic control, and cancer risk. *European Journal of Cancer Prevention.* Epub 2013 Aug 19.

Patterson E, Larsson SC, Wolk A, Åkesson A. Association between dairy food consumption and risk of myocardial infarction in women differs by type of dairy food. *Journal of Nutrition.* 2013 Jan; 143(1):74–9. doi: 10.3945/ jn.112.166330. Epub 2012 Nov 21.

Pereira MA, Jacobs DR, Van Horn L, Slattery ML, Kartashov AI, Ludwig DS. Dairy consumption, obesity, and the insulin resistance syndrome in young adults: the CARDIA Study. *Journal of the American Medical Association.* 2002; 287(16):2081–89. doi:10.1001/jama.287.16.2081.

Qin LQ, Xun P, Bujnowski D, Daviglus ML, Van Horn L, Stamler J, He K; INTERMAP Cooperative Research Group. Higher branched-chain amino acid intake is associated with a lower prevalence of being overweight or obese in middle-aged East Asian and Western adults. *Journal of Nutrition.* 2011 Feb; 141(2):249–54. doi: 10.3945/jn.110.128520. Epub 2010 Dec 15.

Rossi M, Turati F, Lagiou P, Trichopoulos D, Augustin LS, La Vecchia C, Trichopoulou A. Mediterranean diet and glycaemic load in relation to incidence of type 2 diabetes: results from the Greek cohort of the population-based European Prospective Investigation into Cancer and Nutrition (EPIC). *Diabetologia.* 2013 Nov; 56(11):2045–13. doi:10.1007/s00125-013-3013-y. Epub 2013 Aug 22.

Rouse M, Carlson O, Egan JE. Resveratrol and curcumin enhance pancreatic and beta-cell function by inhibiting phosphodiesterase activity. *Endocrine Reviews.* 2013; 34(03):mon–819.

Salas-Salvadó J, Bulló M, Babio N, Martínez-González MÁ, Ibarrola-Jurado N, Basora J, Estruch R, Covas MI, Corella D, Arós F, Ruiz-Gutiérrez V, Ros E; PREDIMED Study Investigators. Reduction in the incidence of type 2 diabetes with the Mediterranean diet: results of the PREDIMED-Reus nutrition intervention randomized trial. *Diabetes Care.* 2011 Jan; 34(1): 14–19. doi: 10.2337/dc10-1288. Epub 2010 Oct 7.

Schellekens H, Finger BC, Dinan TG, Cryan JF. Ghrelin signalling and obesity: at the interface of stress, mood and food reward. *Pharmacology & Therapeutics.* 2012 Sep; 135(3):316–26. doi: 10.1016/j.pharmthera.2012.06.004. Epub 2012 Jun 27.

Schernthaner G, Schernthaner GH. Diabetic nephropathy: new approaches for improving glycemic control and reducing risk. *Journal of Nephrology.* 2013 Nov–Dec; 26(6):975–85. doi: 10.5301/jn.5000281. Epub 2013 Jun 14.

Shen J, Obin MS, Zhao L. The gut microbiota, obesity and insulin resistance. *Molecular Aspects of Medicine.* 2013 Feb; 34(1):39–58. doi: 10.1016/j.mam.2012.11.001. Epub 2012 Nov 16.

Siri-Tarino PW, Sun Q, Hu FB, Krauss RM. Saturated fat, carbohydrate, and cardiovascular disease. *American Journal of Clinical Nutrition.* 2010 Mar; 91(3):502–9. doi: 10.3945/ajcn.2008.26285. Epub 2010 Jan 20.

Siriwardhana N, Klaupahana NS, Cekanova M, LeMieux M, Greer B, Moustaid-Moussa N. Modulation of adipose tissue inflammation by bioactive food compounds. *The Journal of Nutritional Biochemistry.* 2013 Apr; 24(4): 613–23.

Sluijs I, Forouhi NG, Beulens JW, van der Schouw YT, et al; InterAct Consortium. The amount and type of dairy product intake and incident type 2 diabetes: results from the EPIC-InterAct Study. *American Journal of Clinical Nutrition.* 2012 Aug; 96(2):382–90. Epub 2012 Jul 3.

Takikawa M, Kurimoto Y, Tsuda T. Curcumin stimulates glucagon-like peptide-1 secretion in GLUTag cells via Ca/calmodulin-dependent kinase II activation. *Biochemical and Biophysical Research Communications.* 2013; 435:165–70.

Tremblay A, Gilbert JA. Milk products, insulin resistance syndrome and type 2 diabetes. *The Journal of the American College of Nutrition.* 2009 Feb; 28(suppl 1):9lS–102S.

Wang W, Xie Z, Lin Y, Zhang D. Association of inorganic arsenic exposure with type 2 diabetes mellitus: a meta-analysis. *Journal of Epidemiology & Community Health.* 2014 Feb 1; 68(2):176–84. doi: 10.1136/jech-2013-203114. Epub 2013 Oct 16.

Wedick NM, Pan A, Cassidy A, Rimm EB, Sampson L, Rosner B, Willett W, Hu FB, Sun Q, van Dam RM. Dietary flavonoid intakes and risk of type 2 diabetes in US men and women. *American Journal of Clinical Nutrition.* 2012 Apr; 95(4):925–33. doi: 10.3945/ajcn.111.028894. Epub 2012 Feb 22.

Wimalawansa SJ. Visceral adiposity and cardiometabolic risks. *Res Reports Endocrine Disorders.* 2013; 3:17–30.

Xiao Q, Arem H, Moore SC, Hollenbeck AR, Matthews CE. A large prospective investigation of sleep duration, weight change, and obesity in the NIH-AARP Diet and Health Study cohort. *American Journal of Epidemiology.* 2013 Dec 1; 178(11):1600–10. doi: 10.1093/aje/kwt180. Epub 2013 Sep 18.

Yang Z-H, Miyahara H, Hatanaka A. Chronic administration of palmitoleic acid reduces insulin resistance and hepatic lipid accumulation in KK-Ay mice with genetic type 2 diabetes. *Lipids in Health and Disease.* 2011; 10:120.

Zamora-Ros R, Forouhi NG, Sharp SJ, González CA, Buijsse B, Guevara M, et al. The association between dietary flavonoid and lignan intakes and incident type 2 diabetes in European populations: the EPIC-InterAct study. *Diabetes Care.* 2013 Dec; 36(12):3961–70. doi: 10.2337/dc13-0877. Epub 2013 Oct 15.

ACKNOWLEDGMENTS

Our heartfelt thanks to our excellent agent, Carole Bidnick, who made sure we had the opportunity to express our professional beliefs about this huge public health problem.

Kudos to editor par excellence Julie Bennett. We were so lucky to benefit from her hands-on talents even as she juggles all her responsibilities as editorial director for Ten Speed's outstanding list. She worked tirelessly to help us make this the best book it could be, and we are most grateful.

Thanks also to the other professionals at Ten Speed Press and Penguin Random House who threw their support behind *The Diabetes Solution*: Aaron Wehner, Hannah Rahill, David Drake, Carisa Hays, Kristin Casemore, Michele Crim, Kara Van de Water, Lorraine Woodcheke, Daniel Wikey, Betsy Stromberg, and Anitra Alcantara. And to our persevering publicist, Mary "Sunshine" Lengle.

INDEX

F

Fajitas, Steak, 189–90
Falls prevention, 229
Fats
    functions of, 16
    "good" and "bad," 104–7
    saturated, 121
    trans, 125–26
    See also Body fat
Fiber, 16, 108, 131
Finances, stress from, 239
Fish, 112, 168
    Chinese-Style Steamed Black
      Bass with Ginger, Leeks, and
      Mushrooms, 170
    Cod-Corn Chowder, 161
    Flounder with Almonds and
      Lemon Butter, 168
    Moroccan Fish Tagine en
      Papillote, 175–76
    Salmon Cupcakes with Cucumber-
      Yogurt Sauce, 171–72
    Salmon-Stuffed Cabbage with
      Savory Lentils, 169
    Smoked Trout in Endive
      Spears, 149
    Spice-Rubbed Salmon Kebabs with
      Minted Yogurt Sauce, 176–77
    Tilapia in Tomato-Caper Sauce
      with Kalamata Olives, 173
Flight-or-fight response, 236
Flour, 124, 125
Folate, 72
Foods
    to avoid, 110–11, 124–27
    good and bad, 104
    interactions between, 105–6
    to limit, 121–23
    organic, 15, 139
    super-, 105
    See also Blood Sugar Budget; Diet;
      individual foods
Foot care, 65
FPG (Fasting Plasma Glucose) test,
    23–24
Framingham Heart Study, 106–7
Fried foods, 125–26
Frittatas, 156–57

Fruits
    dried, 123
    recommended, 117, 119, 134
    See also individual fruits

G

Gastric bypass surgery. *See* Bariatric
    surgery
Gastroparesis, 64
Gestational diabetes (GDM), 93–99
GFR (glomerular filtration rate),
    60–61
Ghrelin, 241
Glucagon, 19
Gluconeogenesis, 241
Glucose, 17, 18, 19. *See also* Blood
    sugar levels; Sugar
Glycemic index and glycemic load, 108
Glycogen, 18
Goulash, Hungarian Pork and
    Sauerkraut, 192–93
Grains, 117, 119, 134, 208. *See also*
    individual grains
Granola, Crunchy Cranberry, 154
Griddle Cakes, Whole Grain, 154–55
Gym, alternatives to, 230

H

Half-and-half, 124
Ham
    Turnip and Mustard Green
      Soup with Pinto Beans and
      Ham, 166
    See also Prosciutto
Hazelnut Torte, 220
Heart attacks, 61–62
Heart rate, maximum, 228
Hemoglobin A1C (Hgb-A1C), 14–15,
    23, 26–30, 35
Hydration, 135
Hyperglycemia, 9, 13, 54–55
Hypoglycemia, 14–15, 55–57

I

Incretin, 247
    mimetics, 87
Infections, nonhealing, 64–65

Inflammation, 15, 40, 108, 139
Insulin
  avoiding spikes in, 110, 111
  injections, 87–89, 91
  production of, 11, 19
  pumps, 88, 90
  resistance, 11, 97, 108, 236
  role of, 19
Integrative medicine, 235–36, 253–54
Isometrics, 232

J

Joe's Special One-Skillet Meal,
  187–88

K

Kale
  Asian Quinoa with Spinach and
    Mushrooms, 212
  Green Chicken Chili with White
    Beans, 180
  Italian Minestrone, 167
  Kale Salad with Sweet Potato
    "Croutons," 203
  Quinoa with Cranberries and
    Kale, 212–13
  Strawberry Magic Smoothie, 158
  Zesty Kale Dip, 145
Ketoacidosis, 11, 55
Ketones, 55
Keys, Ancel, 107
Kidney disease, 8, 13, 30, 59–61
Kiwi, Pecan Meringue Torte with
  Berries and, 218

L

Lactic acid, 231
Lamb
  Lamb and Vegetable Curry, 194
  Middle Eastern Lamb and
    Eggplant Stew with Chickpeas
    and Tomatoes, 193
Lap-band surgery. *See* Bariatric
  surgery
Lemons
  Blueberry Lemon Frost, 159
  Lemon Cream, 162

Lemony Escarole and Rice
  Soup, 164
Lemony Stir-Fried Brussels
  Sprouts, 204–5
Lentils
  Salmon-Stuffed Cabbage with
    Savory Lentils, 169
  Savory Lentils with Mushrooms
    and Dill, 205

M

Mango Smoothie, Tropical, 160
Mayonnaise, 121
  Aioli (aka Garlic Mayonnaise)
    with Spring Vegetables, 144
Meals
  number of, 131
  planning, 127–31
  skipping, 137–38
Meat
  fatty cuts, 125
  nutrition and, 189
  portion size for, 132, 137
  processed, 112, 125
  TMAO in, 112
  See also Beef; Lamb; Pork
Medications
  for diabetes, 78–91
  for erectile dysfunction, 70–71
  managing, 252
  mistrust of, 76
  for prediabetes, 43
  for sleep, 242–43
Mediterranean diet, 107, 109, 113,
  136
Meglitinides, 82–83
Menus, sample, 128–30
Metabolic syndrome, 41–42, 108
Metformin, 15, 34, 73, 78, 80–81,
  97–98
Milk, 104–5, 117, 136
Minestrone, Italian, 167
Mushrooms
  Asian Quinoa with Spinach and
    Mushrooms, 212
  Balsamic Chicken with
    Mushrooms and Sweet Red
    Pepper, 178

Pork, 112
Hungarian Pork and Sauerkraut
Goulash, 192–93
Mustard-Crusted Pork
Tenderloin with Roasted
Cabbage and Fennel, 191–92
See also Ham; Prosciutto
Potatoes, 122
Cod-Corn Chowder, 161
Italian Minestrone, 167
Italian Vegetable Frittata, 156–57
Roasted Winter Vegetables, 204
Smoked Turkey Hash, 153
Prediabetes
blood sugar levels and, 12, 37–38
body weight and, 39–41
characteristics of, 37–38
dealing with, 2–3, 38–39, 42–51
definition of, 1
diagnosing, 23–30, 39
metabolic syndrome and, 41–42
prevalence of, 7, 38
undiagnosed, 38
Processed foods, 125–26
Prosciutto
Eggplant Stuffed with Mozzarella
and Prosciutto in Basil Tomato
Sauce, 200–201
Stuffed Turkey Breast, 183
Protein
in beans, 135–36
in the Blood Sugar Budget, 117,
136–37
excess, 113
functions of, 16
sources of, 113, 120, 136–37
Psyllium, 45

Q

Quinoa
Asian Quinoa with Spinach and
Mushrooms, 212
Quinoa with Cranberries and
Kale, 212–13

R

Radicchio, Roasted Cauliflower and,
in Anchovy-Garlic Sauce, 200

Rajas, 190
Raspberries
A Berry Berry Morning, 159
Pecan Meringue Torte with Kiwi
and Berries, 218
Resistance training, 231–32
Retinopathy, 13, 58
Rice, 122
Asparagus Risotto, 211
Lemony Escarole and Rice
Soup, 164

S

Salads
Asian Slaw, 195–96
Dilled Barley Salad with Corn and
Edamame, 208–9
Jalapeño Cabbage Salad, 197
Kale Salad with Sweet Potato
"Croutons," 203
Middle Eastern Chopped Salad, 197
Provençal Vegetable Salad with
Chickpeas and Basil, 206
Tabbouleh, 216
Thai Confetti Slaw, 187
Thai Grilled Beef Salad, 190–91
Wheat Berry Salad, 210
Sandwiches, Cucumber, with Goat
Cheese and Arugula, 146
Sauces
Basil Tomato Sauce, 201
Cucumber-Yogurt Sauce, 172
Lemon Cream, 162
Minted Yogurt Sauce, 177
Sauerkraut Goulash, Hungarian Pork
and, 192–93
Seeds, 117, 120, 136
Sesame-Ginger Dressing, 195–96
Shrimp
Spanish Garlic Shrimp, 172–73
Tuscan Shrimp with Cranberry
Beans, 174
Slaws, 187, 195–96
Sleep, 50, 235, 241–44
Smoking, 50–51, 68, 69–70
Smoothies, 158–60
Snacks, 111, 144–49
Sodas, diet, 126

Type 2 diabetes
 aging and, 12
 blood sugar levels and, 11–12
 cardiovascular disease and, 1, 7, 13
 as cause of death, 2, 7
 complications from, 13–14, 53–73
 diagnosing, 14–15, 22–30
 dismissal of, 8–9, 10
 gestational diabetes and, 94
 impact of, 7–8, 254
 insulin resistance and, 11
 monitoring, 35–36
 nutrition and, 15–20
 obesity and, 12, 31
 prevalence of, 2, 7, 12
 risk factors for, 7–8, 33
 screening for, 30–33
 sleep and, 235, 241–44
 stress and, 235, 236–41
 symptoms of, 13, 30
 treating, 2–3, 20, 34–35, 73–74,
  75–91, 251–54
 type 1 vs., 10–11

V
Vegetables
 leafy green and nonstarchy, 117,
  119, 132–33
 starchy and sugary, 121–22
 See also individual vegetables
Vision, blurred, 58
Vitamins
 B$_6$, 72
 B$_{12}$, 72
 D, 45
 folate, 72

W
Walking, 99, 228–30
Walnuts
 Baked Apples with Walnuts and
  Maple Syrup, 217
 Black Bean and Veggie Burgers
  with Bulgur and Oats, 214
 Roasted Eggplant and Walnut
  Dip, 147
Water, 135
Weight lifting, 231–32
Weight loss
 through bariatric surgery, 245–49
 blood pressure and, 238, 252
 Blood Sugar Budget and, 139
 blood sugar levels and, 237–38, 252
 counseling, 238
 exercise and, 231
 for gestational diabetes prevention,
  98–99
 prediabetes and, 46–49
 setting goals for, 47
 as sign of diabetes, 31
 See also Bariatric surgery; Obesity
Wheat Berry Salad, 210
Wine, 123
Work problems, 240

Y
Yoga, 231, 232
Yogurt Sauce, Minted, 177

Z
Zucchini. *See* Squash